Virology Research Progress

Hepatitis B

New Research

VIROLOGY RESEARCH PROGRESS

Additional books in this series can be found on Nova's website under the Series tab.

Additional E-books in this series can be found on Nova's website under the E-book tab.

PUBLIC HEALTH IN THE 21ST CENTURY

Additional books in this series can be found on Nova's website under the Series tab.

Additional E-books in this series can be found on Nova's website under the E-book tab.

VIROLOGY RESEARCH PROGRESS

HEPATITIS B

NEW RESEARCH

JEFFREY T. COX
AND
DEDRICK I. OWEN
EDITORS

NOVA BIOMEDICAL

New York

For permission to use material from this book please contact us:
Telephone 631-231-7269; Fax 631-231-8175
Web Site: http://www.novapublishers.com

Library of Congress Cataloging-in-Publication Data

LCCN: 2012937528

ISBN: 978-1-62081-846-6

Published by Nova Science Publishers, Inc. † New York

Contents

Preface

Hepatitis B virus (HBV) infection is a problem of global health importance and represents a significant cause of morbidity and mortality worldwide. HBV can be transmitted parenterally, sexually and perinatally. Despite progress on prophylaxis, diagnostic and treatment of HBV infection, it remains one of the major causes of chronic liver disease, cirrhosis or hepatocellular carcinoma. This book presents a compilation of current research including such topics as Hepatitis B and dialysis; Hepatitis B virus infection among middle school students in South Brazil; genotyping and management of chronic Hepatitis B; the risk assessment for Hepatitis B infection and its role in hepatocellular carcinoma; and silencing Hepatitis B virus replication with antiviral Pri-Mir shuttles generated from liver-specific Pol II promoters.

Chapter I - Hepatitis B virus (HBV) is 50 to 100 times more contagious than Human Immunodeficiency Virus (HIV). Globally, 2 billion people have been infected with HBV, 350 million have chronic infection, and approximately 600,000 deaths are recorded every year due to consequences of hepatitis B infection. 25% of adults who contract infection during their childhood eventually die from hepatocellular carcinoma or liver cirrhosis. Although an effective vaccine is available to prevent HBV infections, the number of chronic cases and deaths are still on count. Chemotherapy for HBV infection includes limited number of effective drugs. The available nucleoside analogs e.g., lamivudine and hepsera, have excellent antiviral activity, however, viral rebound and flare-up after cessation of therapy, and development of resistance after long-term use are major clinical limitations. IFN-α therapy does not provide very promising response in HBV infected patients. Several promising new chemotherapeutic and immunotherapeutic approaches and combinations of existing drugs are being investigated in various preclinical and clinical studies. It can be forecasted that the ongoing research would lead to new, effective and short-term treatment regimens, without the development of resistance and viral rebound.

Chapter II - There has been a substantial decrease in the incidence of hepatitis B virus (HBV) infection among dialysis populations, largely due to improvements in infection control procedures and the widespread implementation of HBV vaccination. However dialysis patients remain at increased risk of HBV infection acquisition because of their increased exposure to blood products, shared dialysis equipment, frequent breaches of skin, and immunodeficiency. The rate of serum hepatitis B surface antigen (HBsAg) seropositivity in patients on maintenance haemodialysis in the developed world is low; although sporadic outbreaks of acute HBV infection continue to occur in this setting. The natural history of HBV among patients undergoing long-term dialysis remains unclear. HBV-related liver disease is frequently asymptomatic in dialysis patients and liver-related mortality in this population is very low. There are no rigorously controlled trials for treatment of hepatitis B with either interferon or lamivudine therapy in dialysis patients currently available. This chapter reviews the epidemiology, modes of transmission, diagnosis, prevention and treatment of HBV. Strategies to improve vaccination response, new therapeutic options and selection of patients for therapy will be specifically discussed.

Chapter III - Strong systemic and long lasting immune response becomes prerequisite when vaccination against hepatitis B is desired. Currently used vaccine for hepatitis B contains one of the viral envelope proteins hepatitis B surface antigens (HBsAg). This strongly evokes humoral immune response and hence protects against the infection. However, cellular immune response which is one of the most important bio-responses that contributes in virus elimination from infected hepatocytes cannot be achieved using conventional vaccine. Although, adjuvant based vaccination develop strong humoral response but it remains ineffective in generating desired cellular response. Therefore, to develop a novel and effective vaccine against hepatitis B several strategies including use of carriers based adjuvant system, development of surface functionalized novel antigen carriers and mucosal immunization etc. have been explored. This article describes recent advances in developing novel drug delivery systems based vaccine against hepatitis B.

Chapter IV - At least two billion people worldwide are estimated to have exposure to hepatitis B infection. Forty-five percent of these exposures occur in areas of high endemicity such as Central and South-East Asia, sub-Saharan Africa, and the Amazon Basin, where population prevalence of hepatitis B is greater than 8% and lifetime risk of infection – occurring primarily during childhood – is greater than 60%. A further 43% of exposures occur in areas with 2-7% prevalence, where lifetime risk ranges between 20 and 60%. In contrast, areas of low prevalence, which include the United States, Western Europe, Australia, and parts of South America, account for the remaining 12% of exposures, where prevalence is less than 2%, with exposures occurring largely in adulthood [1].

Chapter V - *Introduction.* Hepatitis B virus (HBV) infection is still a major public health problem in Brazil. It is estimated that at least 15% of the population has been exposed to HBV. Hepatitis B is unequally distributed throughout the country, as a result of the wide territory and socioeconomic differences. Hepatitis B vaccination in South Brazil began in 1993, limited to children younger than 4 years of age. Currently, it is recommended in a three-dose schedule beginning at birth. Vaccination against HBV is also available for unvaccinated persons up to 29 years. *Objectives.* The aim of this study was to determine the prevalence of hepatitis B markers of infection and immunity among middle school students in the state of Santa Catarina, Brazil. *Patients and methods.* This comprehensive cross-sectional seroprevalence study included 2,044 volunteers aged 10 to 16 years old in five major cities of the state. From 2008 to 2009 blood samples were obtained from all enrolled subjects and stored at –20ºC. HBsAg, anti-HBc and anti-HBs serologies were performed using automated microparticles enzymatic immunoassay (Abbott®, AxSYM System). Previously published results will be analyzed along with new data. *Results.* The overall prevalence of present or past HBV infection in the studied population was 0.9% (18 subjects). Eighty eight percent (88%) of all adolescents had detectable anti-HBs titers and 11% presented susceptibility to HBV infection, with no seromarkers for HBV. *Conclusion.* This study found a very low prevalence of HBV markers of infection and a great percentage of immunity, demonstrating the success of the vaccination program against hepatitis B in the state. These findings preindicate a very optimistic situation as to HBV infection and its consequences in the future for this population. With this continuous decrease in rates of HBV, public health resources could be redirected from treating HBV-related conditions to treating other diseases that cannot be so easily prevented.

Chapter VI - A number of risk factors appear to play a role in hepatocellular carcinoma (HCC), hepatitis B infection being one of the most important. Hepatitis B surface antigen (HBsAg) is the hallmark of hepatitis B virus (HBV) since it is the best and most reliable diagnostic marker. However, since most studies do not rely on longitudinal observations but mostly on cross-sectional studies little is known on time changes in those markers and their incidence. Chronic inflammation and cytokines are key determinants in the development of fibrosis and liver cell proliferation. Integration of HBV DNA into host cellular DNA is crucial during HBV chronic infection by disrupting or promoting expression of cellular genes that are important in cell growth and differentiation. In addition, expression of HBV proteins may have a direct effect on cellular functions, and some of these gene products can promote malignant transformation. Several HBV genes have been found in infected tumoral tissues more frequently than others, including truncated pre-S2/S and hepatitis B X genes. The proteins expressed from these integrated genes have been shown to have intracellular activities that may account for their association with HCC, including effects on cellular growth and apoptosis. A major player involved in this form of viral transactivation is the X protein (HBx) that displays pleiotropic functions and has been implicated in the malignant transformation of chronically-infected liver cells. Occult hepatitis B virus infection is characterized by persistence of HBV DNA in HBsAg-negative individuals. There are evidences that occult HBV constitutes a risk factor for the development of HCC and that the mechanisms whereby overt HBV might induce tumor formation are maintained in those atypical HBV infections.

Chapter VII - Chronic infection with hepatitis B virus (HBV) occurs in approximately 6% of the world's population and is often complicated by cirrhosis and hepatocellular carcinoma (HCC). Existing therapy rarely has durable effects and improving treatment to counter the infection remains an important medical priority. Although harnessing the RNA interference (RNAi) pathway to achieve therapeutic HBV gene silencing holds promise, precise regulation of the expression of silencing sequences is critically important for safe application of this approach. Earlier work from our laboratory demonstrated that pri-miR-31- and pri-miR-122-based anti HBV shuttles were capable of potent, safe antiviral activity and can be used in modular multimeric arrangements. To advance this approach, and limit the potential problems caused by extrahepatic expression of anti HBV RNAi activators, these sequences were placed under control of liver specific transcription control elements, viz. the human Factor VIII (FVIII), alpha-1-antitrypsin (A1AT), HBV preS2 and HBV basic core (BCP) promoters. Using a luciferase reporter gene assay optimal liver-specific transcription control was observed with A1AT and BCP regulating sequences. These elements were then incorporated into pri-miR-expression cassettes and were tested for antiviral efficacy in cell culture and a murine model of HBV replication. Results showed that silencing of HBV replication was achieved. Importantly there was no evidence for disruption of endogenous miR function, which is a significant advantage over use of stronger and constitutively active RNA polymerase (Pol) III promoter RNAi expression cassettes. The use of anti HBV pri-miR shuttles in the context of liver-specific Pol II promoters is likely to have usefulness for therapeutic HBV knockdown, and should also have general applicability to silencing of pathology causing genes in the liver.

In: Hepatitis B: New Research
Editors: J. T. Cox and D. I. Owen
ISBN 978-1-62081-846-6

Chapter I

Chemo - and Immunotherapeutic Approaches for the Treatment of Hepatitis B Virus Infection

***Neeraj Shakya*[1]*, Babita Agrawal*[2] *and Rakesh Kumar*[1,*]**

[1]Department of Laboratory Medicine and Pathology, Faculty of Medicine and Dentistry, University of Alberta, Edmonton, AB, Canada
[2]Department of Surgery, Faculty of Medicine and Dentistry, University of Alberta, Edmonton, AB, Canada

Abstract

Hepatitis B virus (HBV) is 50 to 100 times more contagious than Human Immunodeficiency Virus (HIV). Globally, 2 billion people have been infected with HBV, 350 million have chronic infection, and approximately 600,000 deaths are recorded every year due to consequences of hepatitis B infection. 25% Of adults who contract infection during their childhood eventually die from hepatocellular

---

* Address Correspondence to Dr. R. Kumar, Professor - Department of Laboratory Medicine and Pathology. 1-71 Medical Sciences Building. Phone: (780)492-7545, Email: rakesh.kumar@ualberta.ca.

carcinoma or liver cirrhosis. Although an effective vaccine is available to prevent HBV infections, the number of chronic cases and deaths are still on count. Chemotherapy for HBV infection includes limited number of effective drugs. The available nucleoside analogs e.g., lamivudine and hepsera, have excellent antiviral activity, however, viral rebound and flare-up after cessation of therapy, and development of resistance after long-term use are major clinical limitations. IFN-α therapy does not provide very promising response in HBV infected patients. Several promising new chemotherapeutic and immunotherapeutic approaches and combinations of existing drugs are being investigated in various preclinical and clinical studies. It can be forecasted that the ongoing research would lead to new, effective and short-term treatment regimens, without the development of resistance and viral rebound.

Introduction

Hepatitis B, originally recognized as "serum hepatitis" [1], is an infectious and life-threatening liver inflammatory disease caused by a double-stranded DNA virus of *Hepadnaviridae* family [2] known as hepatitis B virus (HBV). Hepatitis B is epidemic in African and Asian regions, and is endemic in China. Approximately 1% of the population in Western Europe and North America is chronically infected with HBV. The disease often leads to chronic condition, which poses high risk of death (600 000/ year) [3] from liver cirrhosis and liver cancer. Transmission of HBV occurs by exposure to infectious blood or body fluids [4]. HBV infections may be categorized as acute-, active chronic- and inactive HBV carriers. HBV reactivation in inactive HBV carriers is a major problem in immunocompromised people, such as individuals infected with HIV, organ transplant recipients, and patients receiving immunosuppressive therapy [5]. According to the World Health Organization (WHO), globally, an estimated 2 billion people have been infected with HBV, and more than 350 million have chronic liver infections [3].

Hepatitis B infection is effectively preventable by current recombinant vaccination in ~95% recipients [6]; however, the 350 million (and counting) chronic patients still need chemotherapy. At present, seven agents, viz. lamivudine (Epivir), telbivudine (Tyzeka), adefovir dipivoxil (Hepsera), tenofovir (Viread), entecavir (Baraclude) and two immune system modulators peginterferon α-2b (Pegintron) and peginterferon α-2a (Pegasys) [7], are available for the treatment of chronic HBV infection. However, current chemotherapy is inadequate due to associated adverse effects, limited efficacy and fast mutation rate (10^{10-11} point mutations per day in individuals with active replication) [8]. Viral rebound, following cessation of prevailing chemotherapy, is another major concern. To resolve these issues, novel chemo/immunotherapeutic interventions to treat HBV patients and to minimize number of morbidity and mortality owing to this pathogen are needed.

In this chapter, we will present an account of novel potential therapeutics, in addition to the prevailing chemotherapeutic and immunotherapeutic approaches.

The Hepatitis B Virus

In 1970, Dane et al identified hepatitis B virions. After 3 years, in 1973, the viral nature of the Dane particles was confirmed by the detection of an endogenous DNA-dependent DNA polymerase within their core. The HBV genome was characterized as partly double stranded circular DNA with only 3200 base pairs, the smallest (42 nm) known DNA virus. [9] The virion has an outer envelope, consisting of the hepatitis B surface antigen (HBsAg) in a lipid bilayer; this lipid bilayer contains the viral envelope proteins and surrounds a nucleocapsid core, enclosing viral genome.

Life Cycle of Hepatitis B Virus

After entry into hepatocytes, HBV envelope is detached and the viral nucleocapsid is transported from the cytoplasm into the nucleus, where the relaxed circular HBV DNA is converted into a double stranded covalently closed circular DNA (cccDNA). The cccDNA is then organized into nucleosomes to form a viral minichromosome, which the cellular RNA polymerase II transcriptional machinery uses as a template for the synthesis of the viral mRNA. [10]

The transcripts are then translated into the viral proteins. The envelope proteins are synthesized and assembled at the ER membranes and then bud into its lumen. The core protein is synthesized in the cytosol and assembled independently with polymerase protein and the pregenomic RNA (3.5 kB) in order to form the nucleocapsids, where the genomic replication takes place. This assembly, encapsidation and reverse transcription process of the pregenomic RNA is initiated by the binding of the viral polymerase to the 5' encapsidation signal, the epsilon (ε) structure, and a secondary loop of the pregenomic RNA. The resulting pregenomic RNA-polymerase complex is encapsidated by core protein dimers to form the nucleocapsids. Subsequently, reverse transcription leads to the synthesis of the complete minus strand HBV DNA that serves as a template for the synthesis of the positive DNA strand. The molecule circularizes, and synthesis of the plus strand DNA reaches about 50-70% of the minus strand length. At this point, the nucleocapsids can either complete the maturation process by entering the endoplasmic reticulum to acquire the viral envelope and be released as infectious virions from the cell or they re-enter the replication cycle via the intracellular conversion pathway ('recycling'), whereby newly replicated DNA is used to amplify the cccDNA pool in the infected cell. The durability and stability of cccDNA is thought to be a key factor in the long-term maintenance of chronic HBV infection and viral rebound after cessation of therapy. [11]

Therapeutic Approaches in Chronic Hepatitis B (CHB) Virus Infection

Two major strategies have been used to treat chronic HBV infection: direct interference with viral replication and modulation of host's immune responses. The replication of the viral genome is catalyzed by the virus encoded HBV polymerase (pol). HBV pol coordinates the assembly of viral nucleocapsids, catalyzes generation of a DNA primer, functions as both reverse transcriptase (RT) and DNA polymerase, and acts as an RNAase H. [12] HBV DNA pol is significantly different than human DNA pol in its substrate and/or inhibitor specificity; it therefore provides an excellent target for antiviral drug design. Most of the nucleoside agents target the HBV pol thereby interfering in multiple viral processes. A number of non-nucleoside inhibitors of HBV have also been investigated; these inhibit viral replication by interfering at several steps DNA replication, nucleocapsid assembly, virus maturation, capsid organization etc. [13-17] In HBV infection, innate and adaptive immune responses play a major role in the outcome of the initial infection. For instance, effective immune responses can result in viral clearance as found in acute-self-limited HBV infection. In contrast, ineffective antiviral immunity can result in progression to chronic infection. [18] Therefore, passive or active immunotherapy providing both innate and/or adaptive immunity against HBV can in principle be envisioned to provide viral clearance.

Current Chemotherapeutic Agents

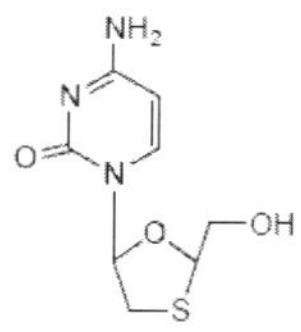

1. Lamivudine (3TC)

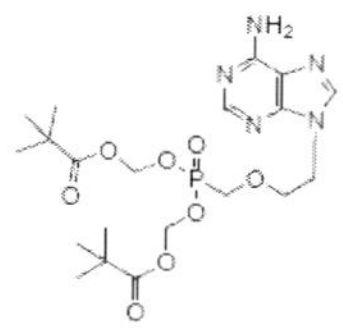

2. Hepsera (Adefovir dipivoxil)

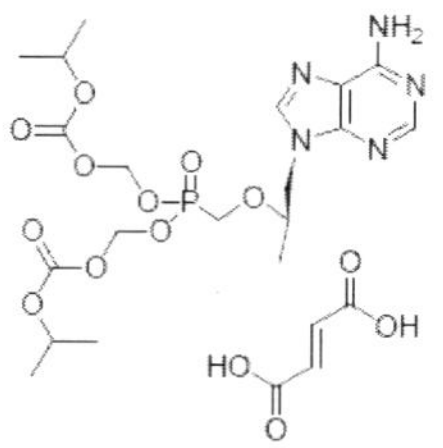

3.Tenofovir disoproxil fumarate (TDF)

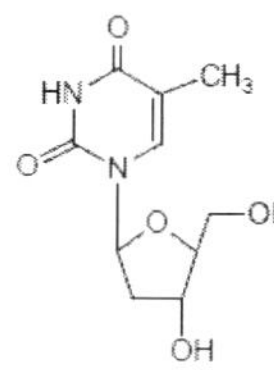

4.Telbivudine

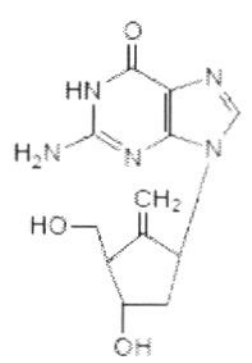

5. Entecavir

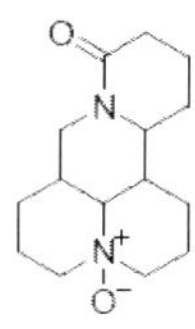

6.Oxymatrine

Chart 1.

Lamivudine (3-TC)

Lamivudine, also known as Epivir or (-)-2',3'-dideoxy-3'-thiacytidine (**1**; Chart 1), is the first and most widely used oral drug, approved in 1998 by FDA for the treatment of chronic HBV infection. It is also indicated as prophylaxis against HBV reactivation in HBsAg-positive, HBeAg-negative individuals with low levels (up to 10^4 IU/mL) of HBV DNA who are to undergo chemotherapy or immunosuppression, particularly for malignancy or transplantation, respectively. [19, 20a] Lamivudine is metabolized within hepatocytes to the active triphosphate form, which then acts as an inhibitor of both reverse transcriptase and DNA polymerase. The absence of hydroxyl group at the 3' position prevents chain elongation by phosphodiester bond formation resulting in chain termination. The potency of lamivudine has been partly attributed to the resistance of its monophosphate to pyrophosphorolytic removal from the viral DNA chain. [20b] It has shown marked suppression of HBV DNA levels, loss of hepatitis B e antigen (HBeAg), seroconversion (defined as HBeAg- negative, antibodies to HBeAg- positive and HBV DNA-negative) and clinical improvements in liver inflammation and histology, in the majority of treated patients. [21, 22] However, after cessation of treatment, relapse has been observed in most of the patients with viremia levels similar to or higher than pre-treatment. Long-term lamivudine therapy results in the development of resistance. The incidence of resistance found are 15-32%, 38%, 56% and 67% at the end of the first, second, third and fourth year of treatment, respectively. [23] Substitutions of methionine to valine or isoleucine at position 204 are responsible for viral resistance during lamivudine therapy. The emergence of resistance is also associated with acute exacerbation of liver disease. [24] It has been found that 20% of the exacerbations may be associated with hepatic functional deterioration, which may be fatal. [25]

In a 5 years treatment study with nucleoside analogs commencing with lamivudine, 96% survival of HBeAg-negative patients was recorded. A recent study revealed that the risk of developing complications such as decompensated cirrhosis and liver-related fatality was significantly reduced in patients with lamivudine therapy than those without therapy. Even in the patients with lamivudine resistance, the long-term complications were lower than those without treatment. Hence, though the risk of hepatitis flare and other side effects associated with lamivudine resistance may limit its use, long-term lamivudine therapy still overweighs no antiviral treatment. [26, 27]

Hepsera (Adefovir Dipivoxil, ADV)

Hepsera (**2**, Chart 1), developed by Gilead Sciences Inc, was approved by the FDA in the year 2002 for the treatment of HBV infection. It is an oral prodrug of an acyclic nucleotide analog of adenosine. After absorption, it is converted to its active form: adefovir. Adefovir is phosphorylated by cellular kinases to the active metabolite adefovir diphosphate, which inhibits HBV DNA pol (reverse transcriptase). Adefovir also acts as a chain terminator when incorporated into viral DNA. In HepG2 2.2.15 cell lines and primary duck hepatocytes infected with duck hepatitis B virus (DHBV), it exhibited EC_{50} values of 0.7 and 0.2 μM, respectively. [28] Adefovir is also effective against lamivudine resistant YMDD mutant HBV strains, although a higher concentration of the drug is required to suppress the M552V mutation.[29] Adefovir was demonstrated to be well tolerated and to reduce serum HBV DNA levels by 4 logs in patients treated for 12 weeks at 30 mg or greater/day. [30] In HBeAg-positive as well as -negative patients adefovir results in sustained decrease in serum HBV DNA level and histologic improvement. In contrast to the low genetic barrier of lamivudine, adefovir has medium genetic barrier to the development of drug resistance. [31] The side effects associated with adefovir therapy are dose related and include nephrotoxicity, lactic acidosis and severe hepatomegaly with steatosis. The cessation of adefovir therapy may result in serious hepatitis.

In clinical trials, after the discontinuation of adefovir, 25% of patients had exacerbations of hepatitis (ALT elevation of 10-fold or greater of the normal levels) and even fatalities. [32]

Tenofovir Disoproxil Fumarate (TDF)

Tenofovir (**3**, Chart 1) is a closely related analog of adefovir dipivoxil. The FDA approved it in the year 2008 for chronic HBV infection. This drug has also been marketed by Gilead Sciences under the trade name Viread. It is a reverse transcriptase inhibitor nucleotide analog. The efficacy of TDF is superior to adefovir in terms of viral suppression, ALT normalization and HBsAg loss after 48 weeks of treatment. [33] According to Woo et al., it was most effective in inducing undetectable serum HBV DNA, ALT normalization, HBeAg seroconversion and HBsAg loss for HBeAg-positive patients. For HBeAg negative patients, TDF was effective in inducing undetectable serum HBV DNA and improving liver histology [34].

In a clinical study, 266 patients with HBeAg positive chronic HBV were randomly assigned to tenofovir (300 mg) or adefovir (10 mg) in a ratio of 2:1.[33, 35] Significantly more patients who received tenofovir achieved HBsAg loss (3 versus 0 percent), ALT normalization (68 versus 54 percent) and HBV DNA level of <400 copies/mL (76 versus 13 percent). In a follow-up report, out of 214 HBeAg positive patients who completed a total of 144 weeks of treatment of TDF, 72% patients had HBV DNA levels <400 copies/mL, while 34% lost HBeAg. [35b] Tenofovir was shown not to be prone to drug-resistance mutations even after 3 years of treatment. [35c] TDF treatment may lead to acute renal impairment in HIV patients [36], however in HBV patients, serum creatinine increase was not significant after 4 years of therapy.

Telbivudine

Telbivudine or L-2'-deoxythymidine (**4**, L-dT; Chart 1), a natural β-L-nucleoside was approved by the US FDA in 2006. It is a potent (EC_{50} = 0.19 μM) and selective inhibitor of HBV replication in HepG2 2.2.15 cells. [37, 38] It acts as a HBV polymerase inhibitor and preferentially inhibits HBV second strand (DNA-dependent) DNA synthesis, in contrast to lamivudine, which preferentially inhibits first-strand (RNA- dependent) DNA synthesis. [39, 40] Telbivudine reduced plasma viremia by up to 8 logs in the woodchuck model of chronic HBV infection at 10 mg/kg/day for 4 weeks. However, HBV DNA was rebounded to pretreatment level after 8 weeks of drug withdrawal. [37] Telbivudine demonstrated no mutagenic, carcinogenic, embryonic or fetal toxic effects in preclinical studies. [41] In a small clinical trial, treatment with telbivudine at 100 to 400 mg/day for 28 days resulted in a 3- to 4-log decrease in HBV DNA levels. [42] HBeAg-positive and HBeAg-negative patients treated with telbivudine had a greater reduction of serum HBV DNA levels than those treated with lamivudine. [43] Like lamivudine, telbivudine also suffers from rapid emergence of drug resistance. Telbivudine resistant mutations are cross-resistant with lamivudine [44], thus it cannot be used for the treatment of patients with proven lamivudine resistance.

Other natural β-L-nucleosides e.g. L-dC (torcitabine), the mono (or di) valine ester of L-dC and L-dA, also exhibited activity against HBV replication *in vitro* and *in vivo*,[37] and are at various stages of clinical development.

Entecavir (Baraclude)

The FDA approved Entecavir (5, Chart 1) in 2005 for the treatment of chronic hepatitis B (CHB) treatment in adults. Entecavir showed EC_{50} of 4 nM against wild type HBV DNA synthesis in human HepG2 2.2.15 cells. The EC_{50} value for entecavir against lamivudine–resistant HBV (rtL 180M, rtM

204V) was 0.010-0.059 μM. Entecavir acts by inhibiting reverse transcriptase, DNA polymerase activities, chain termination and also inhibiting the priming step. [45] Entecavir treatment significantly reduced viral DNA levels (4 to 8 logs) in woodchucks chronically infected with woodchuck hepatitis virus (WHBV) and ducks infected with duck HBV.

Long-term treatment in woodchucks demonstrated that oral weekly dosing of 0.5 mg/kg entecavir maintained viral DNA levels at undetectable levels (<200 copies/mL by PCR) for upto 3 years in 3 of 5 woodchucks. [46] Entecavir has slow rebound of viremia in comparison to lamivudine, which could be partly due to its effect on the cccDNA pool. [47]

In a study of entecavir treatment on chronic HBV patients, 67% of HBeAg-positive patients and 90% of HBeAg-negative patients achieved undetectable serum HBV DNA levels after 48 weeks. [48] A recent study on the relative efficacies, including IFN-therapy and nucleoside analogs in the first 12 months of CHB treatments, showed entecavir as the most effective drug in improving liver histology. [34] Entecavir has high barrier to drug resistance. [49a]

Although entecavir is the most effective of all the anti HBV agents, its use has been limited because of its relatively high cost and serious side effects such as lactic acidosis and hepatotoxicity.

A meta-analysis of 6 studies found that entecavir was more effective than adefovir for treatment-naive HBeAg positive Asian CHB patients. [49b] However, entecavir was minimally effective in patients who had already developed resistance to lamivudine and adefovir. [49c] A meta-analysis showed that entecavir and tenofovir are most effective antiviral drugs for CHB [34].

Oxymatrine

Oxymatrine (**6,** Chart 1), obtained from *Sophora japonica* is used for the treatment of hepatitis B patients in China. [50] Gao et al have reported a host protein heat-stress cognate 70 (Hsc70) involved in HBV replication, as a target for oxymatrine's antiviral activity. Oxymatrine down-regulates hostHsc70 expression at the post-transcriptional level. Oxymatrine is active for wild-type as well as lamivudine and adefovir resistant strains of HBV. It has been reported to be a safe drug.

Monotherapy with oxymatrine orally for 12 months in 17 CHB patients resistant to lamivudine, reduced serum HBV DNAby 96% and HBeAg by

70%, equal to its efficacy in the naïve CHB cohort (n = 20). Liver biopsy showed that oxymatrine treatment decreased Hcs70 mRNA in liver cells, parallel with a reduction of intracellular HBV DNA. Combination of oxymatrine and lamivudine exhibited better anti-HBV effect as compared to lamivudine monotherapy.

The incidence of drug resistance against lamivudine in the combination group was significantly lower than that in the lamivudine only group (1/15 vs. 7/25; p<0.01) [51, 52].

Chemotherapeutic Agents in Pipeline

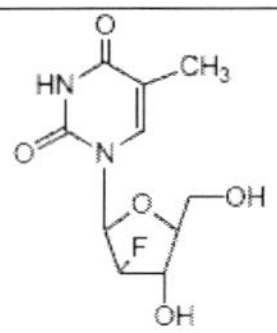 **7**, Clevudine	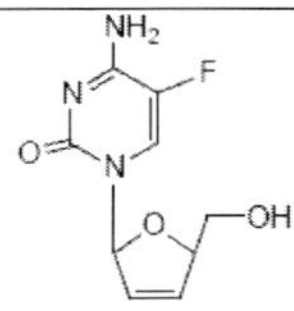 **8**, Elvucitabine
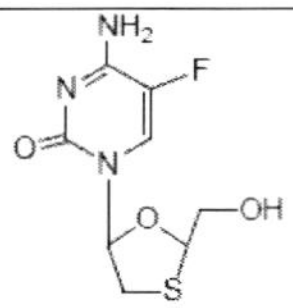 **9**, Emtricitabine	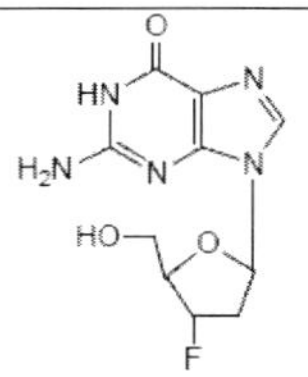 **10**, FLG (MIV-210)
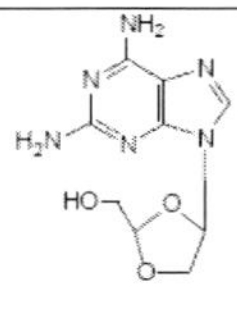 **11**, Amdoxovir	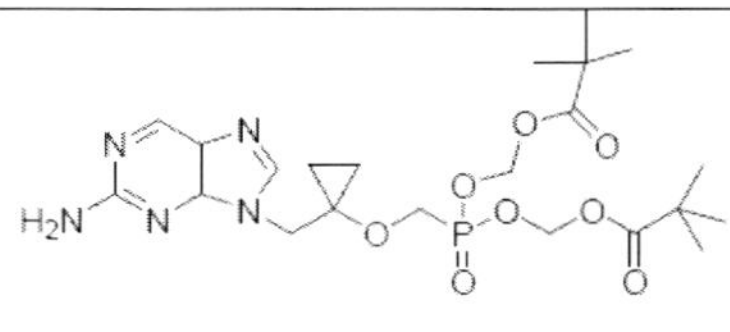 **12**, LB80380
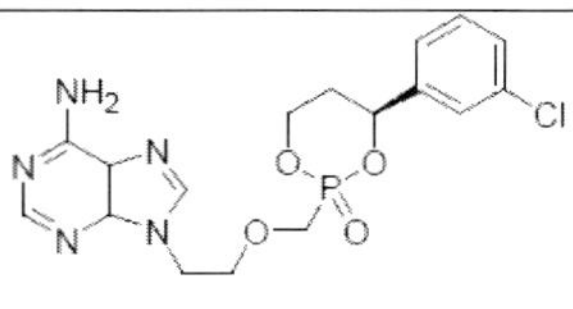 **13**, Pradefovir	

Chart 2.

Clevudine

Clevudine (**7**, L-FMAU; Chart 2) is a potent anti-HBV agent and has been approved in South Korea in 2006 for HBV infection. Clevudine is a potent inhibitor of HBV replication *in vitro* exhibiting an EC_{50} value of 0.08 μM in HepG2 2.2.15 cells. [52, 53] The active triphosphate form of clevudine inhibits the viral DNA polymerase but it is not a chain terminator.

In contrast to other nucleoside agents, it did not exhibit significant rebound in DNA levels after cessation of treatment. [54] Short term oral treatment of chronic DHBV-infected ducklings with L-FMAU at 40 mg/kg/day for 5 days, led to a 72% decrease in viremia levels without any toxicity. [55] In woodchucks chronically infected with WHBV, 10 mg/kg/day of L-FMAU for 12 weeks completely suppressed the viral DNA without any toxicity.

Interestingly, no virus rebound was observed for 24 weeks after cessation of the treatment. Reduction in the cccDNA was also found. [56, 57] In humans, clevudine given at 10, 50, 100 or 200 mg/day for 28 days can reduce the median HBV DNA by 2.5, 2.7, 3 and 2.6 logs, respectively. Clevudine is currently in Phase IV clinical trial. [58]

Elvucitabine

Elvucitabine (**8**, β-L-Fd4C; Chart 2) is a promising drug candidate. It is more potent than lamivudine *in vitro* (EC_{50} = 0.002 μM in HepG2 2.2.15 cells) and *in vivo* in duck and woodchuck model. [37, 59-61] The half-life of its active metabolite, L-Fd4C-TP, is longer than that of lamivudine triphosphate (3TC-TP) in cell culture [62], suggesting that less frequent and lower doses of this agent will still achieve therapeutic efficacy.

Despite its potent efficacy and several fold longer half-life of its metabolite, viremia levels returned to pre-therapy values after cessation of treatment and prolonged treatment was unable to clear intrahepatic viral cccDNA in woodchucks. Furthermore, certain lamivudine-resistant HBV mutations (M5501 and L526M+M550V) are highly cross-resistant to L-Fd4C (EC_{50}> 10 μM). [63, 64] Elvucitabine completed a phase II study for safety and antiviral activity in treatment naive adults with chronic HBV infection. [65] A prodrug of Fd4C, bis(SATE) –L-Fd4CMP, demonstrated more potency and less cytotoxicity than L-Fd4C. [66]

Emtricitabine

Emtricitabine (**9**, FTC; Chart 2) is a 5-fluoro analog of lamivudine. The FDA has not approved it yet for chronic HBV infections. FTC acts by competing as a substrate for HBV polymerase after conversion to its triphosphate by cellular enzymes [67]. It possesses comparable efficacy to lamivudine *in vitro* (EC_{50} = 0.01 to 0.04 μM in HepG2 2.2.15 cells) [37, 59] as well as *in vivo* in both woodchuck and duck models. [68, 69] However, in the woodchuck model, WHBV DNA returned to pretreatment levels 6 days after the cessation of treatment. [70]

In a phase II trial emtricitabine showed HBV DNA suppression in 41% of patients with normalization of serum ALT levels. [71, 72] However, it is cross-resistant with lamivudine-resistant YMDD mutant HBV strains due to its structural similarity to lamivudine. [73-75]

Studies in HIV-1-coinfected patients showed degrees of suppression similar to those noted in patients with HBV infection alone.[76] Emtricitabine is in phase II-IV trials in combination with other drugs [77].

FLG

FLG, a 3'-fluoro-2',3'-dideoxyguanosine (**10**, Chart 2), inhibits wild-type HBV replication in HepG2 2.2.15 cells and also has antiviral potency in the duck model of HBV infection. [78] FLG inhibits wild type DHBV minus-strand DNA synthesis more efficiently compared to lamivudine-triphosphate. The triphosphate of FLG is most likely a competitive inhibitor of dGTP incorporation and a DNA chain terminator.

In Huh7 cells transiently transfected with different HBV constructs, FLG similarly inhibited the replication of wild type, lamivudine-resistant, adefovir-resistant, and lamivudine plus adefovir-resistant HBV mutants. These results were consistent with those obtained in the DHBV polymerase assay using the same drug-resistant polymerase mutants [78].

Thus, FLG can be a suitable agent for the treatment of drug-resistant HBV. A valine prodrug of FLG, MIV-210, has also been shown to inhibit HBV, DHBV and WHBV replication in cell cultures at 2, 0.1 to 0.4 and 1 μM, respectively. [79, 80]

Amdoxovir

Amdoxovir, (-)-β-D-2,6-diaminopurine dioxolane (**11**, DAPD, Chart 2), is a prodrug of dioxolane guanine (DXG), which is converted to parent drug by adenosine deaminase. [81] Amdoxovir has lower antiviral activity compared to lamivudine *in vitro* in HepG2 2.2.15 cells. [59] Amdoxovir acts via inhibiting viral DNA polymerase. Preliminary studies have shown that it is effective against lamivudine-resistant HBV. [82] This compound is currently in phase II clinical trials [83, 84].

LB80380

LB80380 (**12**, Chart 2) is structurally similar to adefovir and tenofovir. It inhibits viral replication by incorporation into the viral DNA. In vitro studies suggest that it has antiviral effect on HBV mutants resistant to lamivudine, adefovir, entecavir and telbivudine. In phase Ib clinical trial it exhibited 3–4.2 log reduction of HBV DNA in treatment-naive patients [85]. In another open labeled phase II dose escalation study in patients with lamivudine-resistant mutations, 12-week treatment of LB30380 exhibited dose-dependent reduction of serum HBV DNA levels. LB80380 is safe and well tolerated up to 240 mg daily dose. [86b] LB80380 is in phase II clinical trial by L G Life Sciences, South Korea [86].

Pradefovir

In 2008, Reddy et al [87] have described pradefovir (**13**, Chart 2), which is a prodrug of adefovir with good oral bioavailability. Tissue distribution studies in rats using radiolabeled materials showed that it metabolizes in the liver and enhances the delivery of adefovir. Pradefovir exhibits a 12-fold improvement in the liver/kidney ratio over adefovir dipivoxil. Its phase II dose-ranging study has been completed. [88]

Other Nucleosides under Investigation

Recently we investigated several lyxofuranosyl, 2'-fluoroxylofuranosyl, 3'-fluoroarabinofuranosyl, and 2'-fluoro-2',3'-didehydro-2',3'-dideoxyribose pyrimidine nucleoside analogues against HBV. Among the compounds examined, 1-(2-deoxy-β-D-lyxofuranosyl)thymine (**14**, Chart 3), 1-(2-deoxy-β-D-lyxofuranosyl)-5-trifluoromethyluracil (**15**), 1-(2-deoxy-2-fluoro-β-D-xylofuranosyl)thymine (**16**) and 2',3'-dideoxy-2',3'-didehydro-2'-fluorothymidine (**17**) were found to possess significant anti-HBV activity against DHBV (EC_{50} values of 4.1, 3.3, 3.8, and 0.2 μM, respectively) and wild-type human HBV in 2.2.15 cells (EC_{50} = 41.3, 33.7, 19.2 and 2.0-4.1 μM, respectively). The compounds **15**, **16** and **17** retained sensitivity against lamivudine-resistant HBV containing a single mutation (M204I). Compound **17** emerged as an effective inhibitor of drug-resistant HBV with an EC_{50} of 4.1 μM. In contrast, 50% inhibition could not be achieved by lamivudine at 44 μM concentration in the drug-resistant strain. These compounds did not display cytotoxicity to the host cells up to the highest concentrations tested. [89]

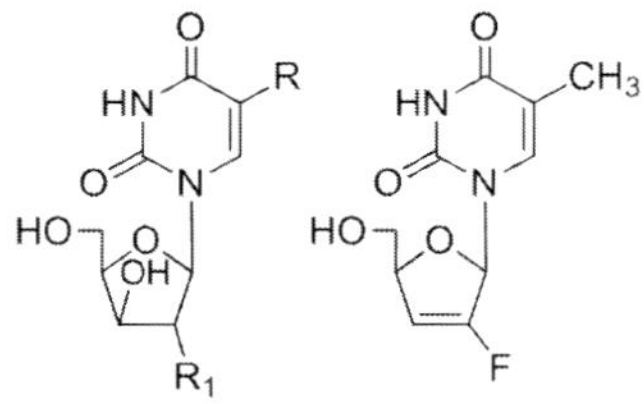

14, R = CH_3, R_1 = H
15, R = CF_3, R_1 = H
16, R = CH_3, R_1 = F
17

We also reported anti-HBV activity ofseveral 5-substituted 3'-fluoro (or chloro) and 2',3'-difluoro 2',3'-dideoxynucleosides (**18-21**) against duck DHBV and human HBV. Among these compounds 5-hydroxymethyl-3'-fluoro-2',3'-dideoxyuridine (**18**) and 1-(3-chloro-2',3'-dideoxy-β-D-*threo*-pentofuranosyl)-5-fluorouracil (**21**) provided the most inhibition [EC_{50} = 1 and 10 μg/mL (DHBV); 5-10 and 10 μg/mL (2.2.15 HBV)] without cytotoxicity. [90]

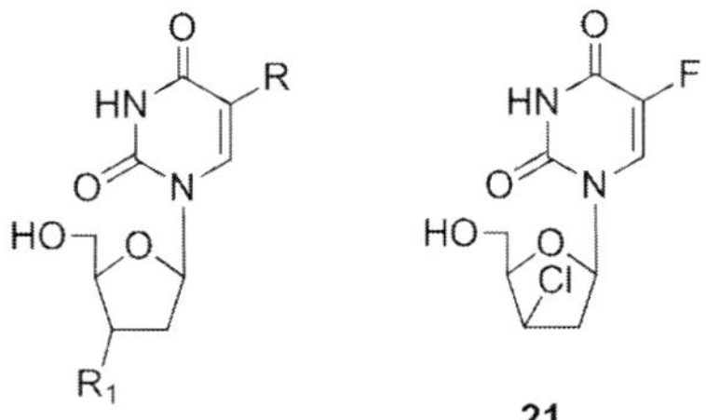

18, R = CH_2OH, R_1 = F
19, R = I, R_1 = F
20, R = CH_3, R_1 = Cl
21

Acyclic Pyrimidine Nucleosides

In our earlier studies, [91] we designed and studied the anti-HBV activity of acyclic pyrimidine nucleosides as a new class of potent and selective inhibitors of DHBV replication. These novel agents were strong inhibitors of HBV replication in primary duck hepatocytes infected with DHBV *in vitro*. The compound 1-[(2-hydroxy-1-(hydroxymethyl)ethoxy)methyl]-5-vinyl uracil (**22**) showed EC_{50} of 0.3-1.0 μg/mL and 1-[4-hydroxy-3-(hydroxymethyl)-1-butyl]-5-(1-azido-2-chloroethyl) uracil (**23**) showed potent activity against DHBV *in vitro* (EC_{50} = 0.31-1.55 μM). [92] In this series, we further investigated acyclic pyrimidines **24**-**26** which exhibited potent and selective anti-DHBV activity at very low concentrations (EC_{50} = 0.01-0.1 μg/mL range). The best compound of this series was found to be 1-[4-hydroxy-3-(hydroxymethyl)-1-butyl]-5-(1-azidovinyl) uracil (**26**) with EC_{50} of 0.01-0.05 μg/mL which is comparable to the reference drug lamivudine (EC_{50} = 0.01-0.05 μg/mL). [93] Later, various 5-, 6- or 5,6-substituted acyclic pyrimidines containing a 1-[(2-hydroxyethoxy)methyl] glycosyl moiety at the N-1 position were synthesized and evaluated for the anti-HBV activity. These analogues showed potent *in vitro* activity in both chronically infected primary duck hepatocytes and a human HBV DNA transfected human hepatoblastoma cell line (HepG2 2.2.15). [94] These compounds also exhibited *in vitro* activity against lamivudine-resistant HBV containing single (M204I) and double (L180M/M204V) mutations. In these studies, we found that 5-halo analogues in particular displayed potent and selective anti-HBV activity.

The most active compound 1-[(2-hydroxyethoxy)methyl]-5-chlorouracil (**27**) of this series exhibited EC_{50} of 0.4-2.2 μM in DHBV *in vitro* and EC_{50} of 4.5-45.4 μM in HepG2 2.2.15 cells, and its activity was quite close to the currently used drug lamivudine against HBV. [94] Further we examined the anti-HBV effect of various 5-substituted acyclic pyrimidine nucleosides containing a 1-[(2-hydroxy-1-(hydroxymethyl) ethoxy)methyl] moiety with a 3'-OH like group, to determine if they have increased affinity for viral DNA polymerase, thus providing improved anti-HBV activity and selectivity. The compounds in which the base moiety was substituted by 5-chloro (**28**), 5-(2-bromovinyl)- (**29**), or 5-bromo-6-methyl- (**30**) groups possess significant activity against DHBV, wild type human HBV (2.2.15 cells), and lamivudine-resistant HBV containing single and double mutations. The most active compound **28** exhibited activity similar to guanine analog ganciclovir against

DHBV and only 10 times lower *in vitro* anti-HBV activity than lamivudine in 2.2.15 cells. [95]

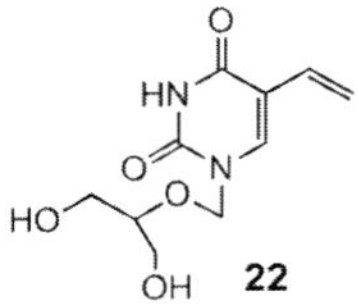
22

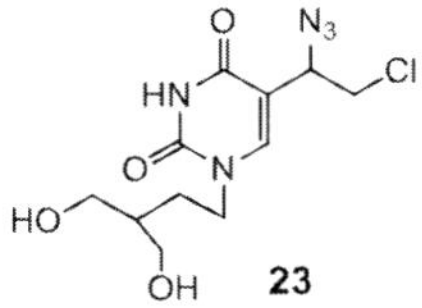
23

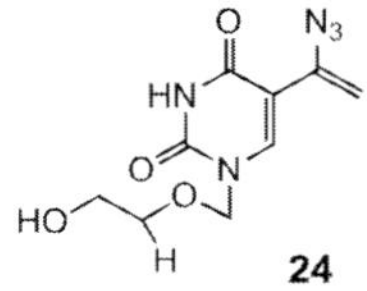
24

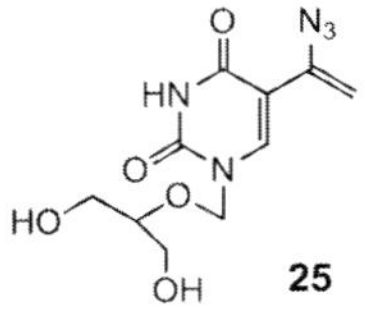
25

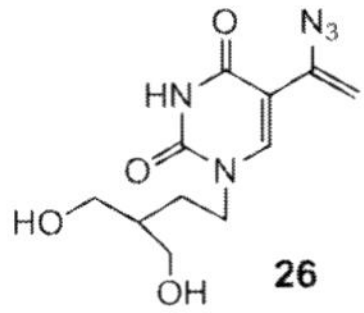
26

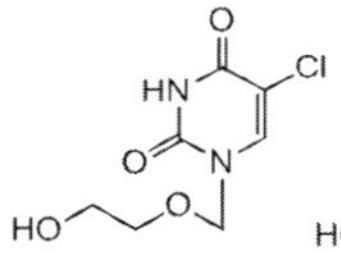
27

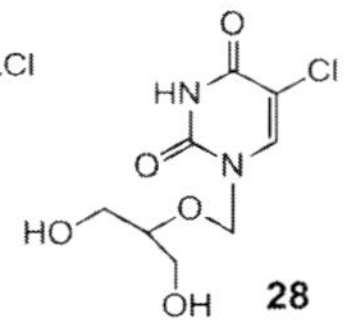
28

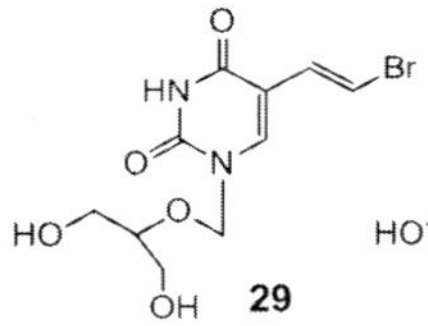
29

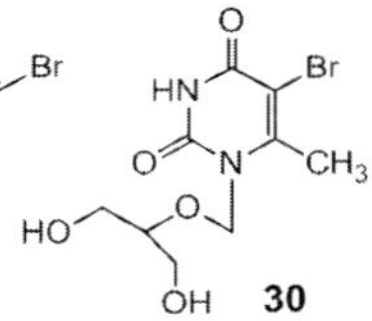
30

Non-Nucleoside Agents in Pipeline

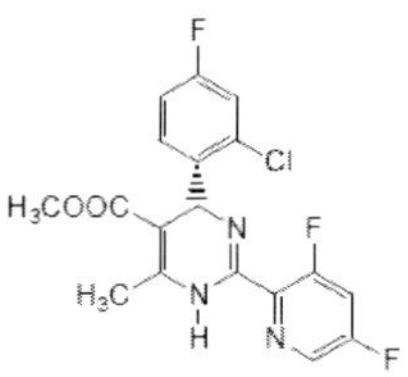 **31**, Bay41-4109	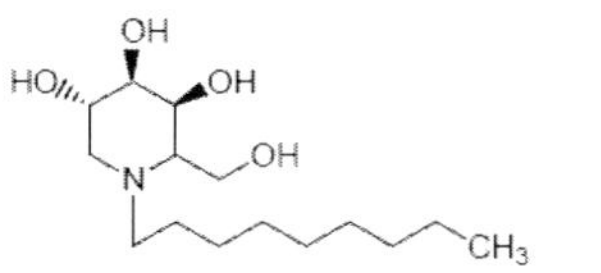 **32**, n- (n-Nonyl)- deoxygalactonojirimycin
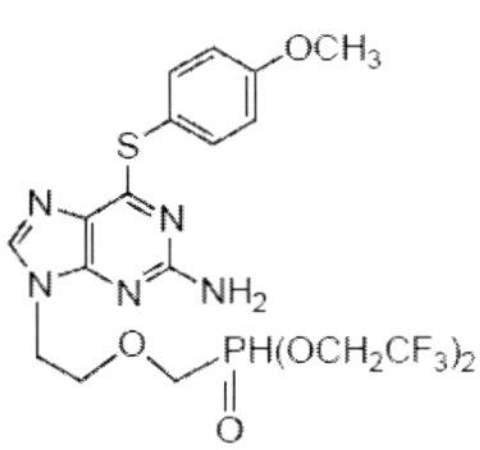 **33**, MCC-478	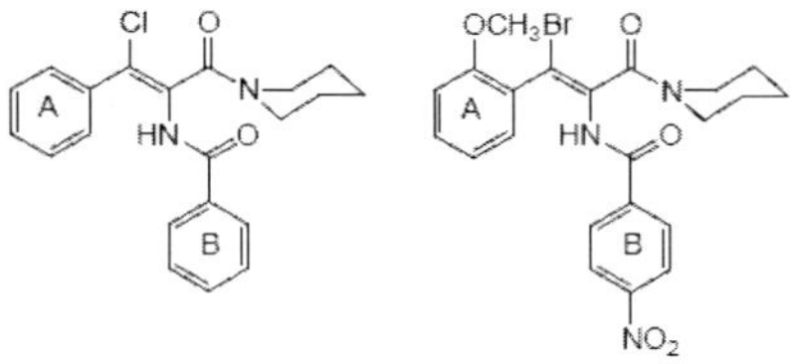 **34**, Phenylpropenamide derivatives AT- 61 and AT- 130

Chart 3.

Bay 41-4109

Bay 41-4109 (**31**, Chart 3) and the congeners Bay 38-7690 and Bay 39-5493 belong to heteroaryldihydropyrimidines (HAP). These non-nucleoside compounds have been reported to inhibit the normal formation of viral nucleocapsids, which are the site of viral DNA replication. In stably transfected HepG2 2.2.15 cells, these compounds showed an EC_{50} of 0.05 μM for the depletion of the viral genome. In the endogenous–polymerase assay, Bay 41-4109 was inactive, suggesting that viral DNA polymerase is not a direct target. Bay 41-4109 also reduces HBV core protein in HepG2 2.2.15 cells. [13] Currently, Bay 41-4109 is under phase I clinical trial by AiCuris, Germany. [85b]

n- (n-Nonyl)- Deoxygalactonojirimycin

n- (n-Nonyl)-deoxygalactonojirimycin (**32**, Chart 3) reduces the amount of HBV DNA produced within the stably transfected HBV producing HepG2 2.2.15 cell lines in culture in a dose dependent manner. It has been shown that this compound either prevents the maturation of HBV nucleocapsids or destabilizes the newly formed nucleocapsids. [14]

MCC - 478

MCC-478 (**33**, Chart 3) is an ester derivative of 2-amino-6-arylthio-9-[bis (2,2,2- trifluoro ethyl)phosphonomethoxyethyl]purine. This compound is highly active and displayed 80 – fold higher activity than lamivudine against HBV. [15] MCC-478 is also active against DHBV and WHBV.

Phenylpropenamide Derivatives AT- 61 and AT- 130

These non-nucleoside compounds (**34**, Chart 3) exhibited EC_{50} values 21.2±9.5 and 2.40±0.92 μM, respectively against wild type human HBV (lamivudine EC_{50}=0.064±0.020 μM). These compounds have no effect on duck HBV, woodchuck HBV or HIV-1. AT-61 is suggested to be very specific inhibitor of HBV replication *in vitro*. The mechanism of action of these compounds is not clear yet. It has been postulated that AT-61 inhibits the packaging of pregenomic viral RNA, which is required for genome replication. [16, 17]

Current Immunotherapeutic Agents

Interferon–α (IFN-α)

This natural glycoprotein possess both antiviral and immunomodulating activities. It inhibits viral entry into hepatocytes and activates viral ribonuclease to inhibit HBV replication. It may also enhance CTL activity, stimulate natural killer cell activity and amplify HLA class I expression on infected cells. [96] Unfortunately, only less than 50% of all chronic HBV patients are eligible for this treatment. Moreover, of the treated, IFN therapy is effective in only those 30 to 40% patients who exhibited high immunoreactivity to HBV as reflected by high alanine aminotransferase (ALT) levels. IFN-α is costly, administered intravenously and has serious side effects such as depression, neurological disturbances, influenza like symptoms, hair loss, leucopenia, thrombocytopenia, thyroid disorders, autoimmune disorders and rashes. [97-99] Currently the most commonly available IFN for HBV is interferon α-2b (Intron-A) although interferon α-2a (Roferon-A) is used in certain hepatitis C cases. [100]

Pegylated interferon (PEG-IFN)

Fast renal elimination and uneven tissue drug distribution adversely affects clinical potency of a therapeutic agent. Pegylation, i.e. attachment of a polyethylene glycol (PEG) moiety to a molecule to slow down the clearance, is a method to address this problem. [101, 102] The attachment of the PEG molecule to IFN-α–2a renders a longer serum half-life (> 100 hours). In the year 2002, PEG-IFNα-2a (Pegasys) was approved by US FDA for the treatment of CHB. [103] PEG-IFNα-2a has been shown to be superior to IFN-α and lamivudine for the treatment of both HBeAg-positive and negative CHB patients. Adverse effects are usually tolerable and similar to the IFN-α. PEG-IFNα-2b (Pegintron) has also been studied and showed the same effect in HBeAg positive and negative CHB patients [104].

Immunoglobulins

Three different immunoglobulin products are commercially available from Biotherapeutics, [105] Nabi [106] and Cangene [107] pharmaceutical companies.

The immunoglobulins have not shown any role in antiviral therapy in chronic HBV patients. Immunoglobulins against HBsAg are used as passive immunization to provide short-term protection following immediate exposure to HBV due to blood transfusion, perinatal exposure of infants, sexual exposure, or household exposure to people with acute HBV infection. In addition to the antibodies, Hepex-B (Cubist Pharm, Cambridge, MA), a combination of two fully human monoclonal antibodies that target HBV surface antigens, was also tested in a phase II trial in post hepatic allograft patients for treatment of end stage liver disease due to hepatitis B infection, however, the study was terminated. [108]

Immunotherapeutic Agents in Pipeline

The overall goal of immunotherapy is to achieve a more enduring virus suppression and/or viral clearance, a goal not readily achieved or even foreseen by available chemotherapeutics alone. The immunotherapeutic agents for the therapy of chronic HBV infection typically fall under two categories. Non-specific immune modulators, which would stimulate non-specific innate immunity consequently stimulating host's adaptive immune responses, and specific therapeutic vaccines, which would stimulate antigen specific adaptive immune responses.

Immunomodulators

REP 9AC

REP 9AC is a nucleic acid-based polymer (NAPs) and is a clinical candidate from REPLICor company. HBsAg plays a role in suppressing the immune system and may allow maintenance of chronic infection. NAPs act by blocking the release of HBsAg by preventing the production of subviral particles from infected hepatocytes, which leads to amelioration of majority of immunosuppression in HBV infection.

NAPs naturally accumulate in the hepatocytes, the location where they are needed the most. It is reported that REP 9AC cleared HBsAg from the blood of seven patients with chronic HBV infection with relatively short treatment regimens.

All of the treated patients showed antibodies to the HBsAg protein and achieved a minimum 1000-fold reduction in virus in their blood. [109a] In another REP 9AC treatment study [109b], 5 of 8 patients cleared serum HBsAg in 7 to 15 weeks. Anti-HBsAg antibodies were observed in 7 of 8 patients.

Six patients showed 3 to 7-log reduction in serum HBV DNA titers after 7-13 weeks of treatment and three of the six were reported to completely control their infection after 20-27 weeks of treatment. REP-9AC has completed Phase II clinical trial. [109a]

Zadaxin (Thymosin-α)

Zadaxin, an immunotherapeutic treatment for CHB, is a synthetic thymosin α-1 that accelerates the replenishment and maturation of thymocytes, stimulates differentiation of T cells, stimulates T cell mediated antibody production and restores T cell function. [110a]

In a phase III clinical trial involving 316 CHB patients, Zadaxin produced a sustained seroconversion (considered to be cured of the virus) in 20% of the treated patients compared to 32% in PEG-IFN treated patients and 16% in lamivudine treated patients. There was significant virologic response even after discontinuation of thymosin-α therapy. In the peripheral blood and liver of the treated patients, IFN-γ producing CD4 T cells, CTLs and NKT cells were increased. Zadaxin appeared to be well tolerated, with few reports of side effects. Zadaxin has completed Phase IV clinical trial [110b].

GS-9620

GS-9620 is an experimental *toll-like receptor 7* (TLR7) agonist and is being currently developed by Gilead. It is 30 times more selective for TLR7 than for TLR8, and has no cross-reactivity with other TLRs. GS-9620 has been found to activate B-cells, T-cells and stimulate IFN production in laboratory and human studies.

It directly activates B-cells and indirectly activates T-cells. GS-9620 induces IFN-α and other immune-modulating cytokines and chemokines at nanomolar concentrations. GS-9620 exhibits antiviral activity against hepatitis B and a related virus in monkeys and woodchucks. In animals, it showed good pharmacokinetics. It had good oral absorption in dogs and was more active by oral route than intravenous administration in monkeys. Lopatin and colleagues tested the safety, pharmacokinetics, and pharmacodynamics of GS-9620 in human volunteers. The double-blind placebo-controlled study included 75 healthy volunteers. Participants received GS-9620 in single ascending doses of 0.3, 1, 2, 4, 6, 8, and 12 mg. GS-9620 was generally safe and well tolerated with single doses through 12 mg.

The most common adverse events were headaches, chills, and fever. There were no serious adverse events. Thus GS-9620 is a promising, oral immunomodulatory agent with low milligram range potency and a good therapeutic window. [111]

Therapeutic Vaccines

DV-601

DV 601 is a therapeutic vaccine, which is comprised of recombinant HBsAg and HBV core antigen (HBcAg). In an intramuscular dose-escalation study in HBV e-antigen positive treatment-naïve or HBV e-antigen negative treatment-tolerant adult patients with CHB, the patients were assessed for the safety and tolerability of DV-601, and for evaluation of virological response and immunogenicity. Only minor transient side effects including fatigue, malaise, chills, and headache were reported. In this study, reductions in HBV DNA, and s and e antigens were recorded in all dose groups. The antibodies to s and e antigens developed in the higher dose groups. An HBV-specific lymphoproliferative response was found in all the patients while HBc-specific IFN-gamma T cell response was recorded in only 2/6 e-antigen positive patients who were administered the highest dose of DV-601. [112a] In a phase 1b clinical evaluation in HBeAg positive and HBeAg negative chronic HBV infected patients in 2010, it was found that DV 601 was safe and well tolerated at all the tested doses.

In this small study, anti-HBe antibodies were elicited in 25% patients (2/8), and anti-HBs antibodies were elicited in 35% (4/14) patients. Among the evaluated 8 patients, two HBeAg positive patients showed HBeAg clearance and only one showed HBsAg clearance [113,114].

Miscellaneous

NOV-205 (BAM-205)

NOV-205 was approved for use in Russia in 2001. It acts through interference with the proteins required for viral replication. Clinical studies in more than 250 Russian hepatitis B patients supported its antiviral effects, where viral load reduced and ALT levels also declined. [115]

Myrcludex B

Myrcludex B is derived from amino acids of the HBV L-protein and is myristoylated at N-terminal. It is an optimized inhibitory HBV pre-S-lipopeptide and inactivates the HBV-preS1-specific receptor and has IC_{50} in picomolar range against HBV and HDV infections. Efficacy studies against different HBV genotypes, and pharmacokinetic and toxicity studies in rats and dogs have been done. It has good pharmacokinetic properties with low toxicity.

Myrcludex B was stable after 24h in serum stability assay. In rats, single dose pharmacokinetic studies following intravenous or subcutaneous administration showed its selective accumulation in the livers 1 h post injection where it could be detected up to 72 h post administration. No mortality or toxicity was observed in single dose 1 and 4 week toxicity studies in rats. Myrcludex-B is under preclinical investigation. [116, 117]

CYT107 or Interleukin 7 (IL-7)

IL-7 is a growth factor produced by stromal cells in the bone marrow and thymus, and by keratinocytes. IL-7 is under development by Cytheris. In randomized open label, controlled multicentre phase I dose escalation study, followed by a phase IIa study, IL-7 has demonstrated safety and sufficient immunological and antiviral activity. [118]

Dendritic Cells (DC) Based Therapy

DC based vaccine therapy, using autologous DCs loaded with recombinant HBsAg have also been examined. [119] In a study, immunization with HBsAg loaded DC induced anti-HBs antibody in all of the healthy volunteers. In a group of CHB patients, immunization with HBsAg loaded DC led to both antiviral and immunomodulatory responses. These results, although highly promising, pose major practical challenges, due to heterogeneity in DC populations and difficulty in producing GMP grade DCs from different patients at various locations.

Combination Therapy

Monotherapy for the HBV infection has been associated with limitations such as development of drug resistance, poor efficacy and/or viral rebound after cessation of therapy. Combination therapy has been proven to be better in other chronic infections such as HIV and tuberculosis. Individual drug in a combination regimen may act at similar and/or different targets of the virus life cycle rendering additive or synergistic effects. Moreover, adjusting the dose of different compounds in combination can minimize adverse effects of an individual component. Further, development of resistant viral mutants can be minimized. Thus, a combination is a better choice for the treatment of chronic HBV infection to achieve more efficient and complete suppression of virus replication.

1. Combination of Chemotherapeutic Agents

Lamivudine Plus Adefovir Dipivoxil

Yatsuji et al [120] investigated the long-term efficacy of adding adefovir dipivoxil to lamivudine as a rescue therapy in 132 patients with lamivudine-resistant chronic HBV infection. After 2 years of treatment, approximately 80% of patients achieved HBV DNA levels of less than 400 copies/ml, and only 1.6% of patients developed adefovir dipivoxil-resistant viral mutations during follow-up. Although these results were promising, the duration of follow-up in the study was too short to draw a definitive conclusion concerning the efficacy of adefovir dipivoxil 'add-on' strategy, as resistance rates could rapidly increase over time.

In a meta-analysis review, six eligible trials (442 patients) were included and evaluated for methodologic quality and heterogeneity. Higher virological response and lower emergence rate of adefovir-associated resistant mutants was recorded in adefovir plus lamivudine compared to adefovir monotherapy ($p < 0.05$).

On the contrary, the rate of seroconversion, HBeAg clearance and ALT normalization were similar between adefovir plus lamivudine and adefovir alone cohorts ($p > 0.05$). Further, switch-to or adding-on adefovir, were both well tolerated. Thus, it was concluded that the combination of adefovir with lamivudine was superior than adefovir alone in inhibiting HBV replication and preventing drug resistance for lamivudine-resistant patients [121].

In another study, efficacy and safety of combined therapy was assessed after 104 weeks of combined treatment and the frequency of persistent lamivudine resistant HBV was analyzed. A total of 78 patients with compensated CHB (Group A) were maintained on either adefovir 10 mg daily ($n = 38$) or placebo ($n = 40$) while continuing lamivudine. The remaining 38 patients were assigned to Group B with decompensated cirrhosis or post liver transplantation and received lamivudine plus adefovir. At week 104, a significant number of patients in Group A on combination therapy (76%) had a decline in serum HBV DNA compared to those receiving lamivudine alone (13%; $p = 0.001$). 52% of Group A patients on combination treatment continued to have the M204V/I HBV mutation compared to 92% receiving lamivudine alone ($p = 0.0013$). Virologic response occurred less frequently in patients expressing persistent lamivudine resistant HBV. At week 104, 87% of patients in Group B, had HBV DNA response (median change from baseline of -5.84 log10 copies/mL). It was concluded that treatment with the combination of lamivudine plus adefovir for 2 years proved effective in lamivudine resistant cases, but in compensated patients, there was a persistently high rate of lamivudine resistant mutants and impaired virologic response [122].

A recent study evaluated the benefit of adefovir alone versus combination therapy with adefovir and lamivudine in maintaining virological, biochemical and histological responses in patients with CHB with or without previous lamivudine therapy. Patients were randomised to receive adefovir and lamivudine (100 mg/daily) or adefovir alone (10 mg/daily) for up to 192 weeks. Study endpoints were (i) maintained virological (HBV DNA <500 copies/mL), biochemical and histological response, (ii) loss of HBeAg and (iii) loss of HBsAg. A total of 41 patients were enrolled, including 31 treatment-naïve and 31 HBeAg-positive patients. 30 Patients continued therapy for 192 weeks. The percentage of patients achieving a combined maintained response was higher in the combination therapy than the monotherapy arm, both at weeks 48 (59% vs. 26%, p = 0.06) and 192 (68% vs. 31%, p = 0.03). At week 192, 76% of the combination and 36% of the monotherapy group had loss of HBeAg (p = 0.03). One patient receiving adefovir cleared HBsAg. Adefovir resistance developed in 6 of 19 (32%) patients in the monotherapy arm. [123]

The data described above are promising for lamivudine plus adefovir dipivoxil combination. Phase III clinical studies are underway for this combination. [124]

Lamivudine Plus Telbivudine

In a randomized, double-blind, multicenter trial the efficacy and safety of telbivudine 400 or 600 mg/day and telbivudine 400 or 600 mg/day plus lamivudine 100 mg/day (Comb400 and Comb600) was compared with lamivudine alone 100 mg/day in 104 HBeAg-positive patients (randomized equiproportional among 5 groups) with compensated CHB.

At week 52, median reductions in serum HBV DNA levels ($\log_{10}$ copies/mL) were recorded as: lamivudine, 4.66; telbivudine 400 mg, 6.43; telbivudine 600 mg, 6.09; Comb400, 6.40; and Comb600, 6.05. Telbivudine monotherapy showed a significant reduction in HBV DNA levels (6.01 vs. 4.57 $\log_{10}$ copies/mL; $p < 0.05$), clearance of PCR-detectable HBV DNA (61% vs. 32%; $p < 0.05$), and normalization of ALT levels (86% vs. 63%; $p < 0.05$) compared with lamivudine monotherapy, with proportionally greater HBeAg seroconversion (31% vs.22%) and less viral breakthrough (4.5% vs. 15.8%). It was found that the combination treatment was not better than telbivudine alone. However, all treatments were well tolerated. [125] This combination is in phase III clinical trial. [126]

Adefovir Dipivoxil Plus Emtricitabine

In a randomized trial, 30 treatment-naive, HBeAg-positive patients were enrolled for combination therapy with adefovir plus emtricitabine (n = 14) or adefovir plus placebo monotherapy (n = 16) for 96 weeks. Treatment was stopped in those with HBeAg seroconversion. At week 96, the median decrease in HBV DNA was higher in the combination group (5.30 vs. 3.98 log10 copies/ ml, p = 0.05). More patients in the combination group had ALT normalization and HBV DNA < 300 copies/ml at week 96 when compared with the monotherapy group [11 of the 14 patients (78.6%) vs. 6 of the 16 patients (37.5%), p = 0.03]. HBeAg seroconversion was similar in the two groups [2/14 (14.3%) vs. 4/16 (25.0%)].

No adefovir or emtricitabine resistance was detected. In those with HBeAg seroconversion, 50.0% had post-treatment relapse. The combination resulted in more potent suppression of HBV DNA over 96 weeks of therapy. [127]

Tenofovir Disoproxil Plus Emtricitabine

In a recent Phase II, double-blind randomized study, 112 patients with CHB and decompensated liver disease were assigned to receive tenofovir/emtricitabine (fixed-dose combination; n = 45), tenofovir (n = 45), or entecavir (n = 22). The primary endpoint was tolerability failure and serum creatinine increase to 0.5 mg/dL from baseline or serum phosphorus <2 mg/dL. Patients with insufficient viral suppression could begin open-label tenofovir/emtricitabine but were considered failures in the interim 48 week analyses for efficacy endpoints. Tolerability failure was infrequent across arms:, 4.4%, and 9.1% in different arms (p 5 0.622). Six patients received liver transplants and six patients died. At week 48, HBV DNA level was <400 copies/mL (69 IU/mL) in 87.8% (tenofovir/emtricitabine), 70.5% (tenofovir), and 72.7% (entecavir) of patients. Proportions with normal ALT were: 57% (tenofovir), 76% (tenofovir/emtricitabine), and 55% (entecavir). HBeAg loss/seroconversion occurred in 21%/21% (tenofovir), 27%/13% (tenofovir/emtricitabine), and 0%/ 0% (entecavir). It was concluded that all treatments were well tolerated in patients with decompensated liver disease due to CHB, with improvement in virologic, biochemical, and clinical parameters. [128]

In another study, 78 CHB patients from five European centers started a tenofovir/emtricitabine combination treatment for virological, biochemical, clinical, and tolerance monitoring. Patients were classified into either treatment simplification (TS), where efficacy of the previous treatment was obtained at tenofovir/emtricitabine initiation, or treatment intensification (TI), where the previous line of therapy had failed. Tenofovir/emtricitabine was given as TS to 24 patients (31%) and as a TI to 54 patients (69%). Median treatment duration was 76 weeks. 48 Weeks after TI, the probability of HBV DNA becoming undetectable was 76%, and reached 94% at week 96. Patients with TS were treated for a median duration of 76 weeks. In this subgroup, no ALT flare-up occurred during follow-up and all patients except one remained HBV-DNA undetectable.

Creatinine levels were optimal in both groups of patients. It was concluded that after a median follow-up of >76 weeks, the tenofovir/emtricitabine combination showed encouraging antiviral efficacy and a good safety profile in all patients with CHB. Long-term tenofovir/emtricitabine assessment was recommended to evaluate possible emergence of resistance. [129] These studies, overall, suggest that combination of tenofovir and emtricitabine can be a promising therapy. This combination is in phase II clinical trial. [130]

Tenofovir Disoproxil Plus Entecavir

In a recent study, 57 patients (37 HBeAg+) with median age of 45 years who had been previously treated with a median of three lines of antiviral therapy (range 1-6), were treated with combination therapy for a median duration of 21 months. Median decline in HBV-DNA level was 3 logs (range 0-8 log; $p<0.0001$), 51/57 patients became HBV-DNA undetectable, after 6 months (95% CI, 4.6-7). The probability for HBV DNA suppression was not reduced in patients with adefovir or entecavir resistance or in patients with advanced liver disease. Viral suppression led to decline in ALT (median 0.7 upper limit of normal range (ULN); range 0.2-2.4; $p = 0.001$). One patient showed HBs-seroconversion while five patients lost HBeAg. Patients with advanced disease did not show clinical decompensation, two patients with cirrhosis and undetectable HBV DNA developed hepatocellular carcinomas. No newly induced renal impairment, lactic acidosis or mortality was observed. The study concluded that the rescue therapy with entecavir and tenofovir in CHB patients harboring viral resistance patterns or showing only partial antiviral responses to preceding therapies was efficient, safe, and well tolerated. [131]

A recent report discussed a case of late onset HBV after a long-term prophylaxis with lamivudine in a patient who underwent *hematopoietic stem-cell transplantation* (HSCT) for non-Hodgkin lymphoma and who was successfully treated with a combination antiviral regimen including entecavir and tenofovir disoproxil fumarate [132].

Another report showed a case of HBV reactivation in a patient with non-Hodgkin's lymphoma following a rituximab-based regimen, and who was successfully treated with a combination antiviral treatment including entecavir and tenofovir disoproxil fumarate. [133]

The above studies reveal that the combination of tenofovir disoproxil plus entecavir is safe and effective. This combination is in phase III clinical trial. [134]

Adefovir Plus Entecavir

In a randomized active-control 52-week trial, 90 patients (with serum HBV DNA >2000 IU/mL) who were previously treated for 24 weeks with lamivudine plus adefovir therapy for lamivudine-resistant HBV, received combination of entecavir plus adefovir (n = 45) or continuation of lamivudine plus adefovir (n = 45) for 52 weeks. The baseline patients' mean serum HBV DNA was 4.60 $\log_{10}$ IU/mL. At week 52, the proportion of patients with serum HBV DNA <60 IU/mL was considerably greater in the entecavir plus adefovir group than in the lamivudine plus adefovir group (n = 13, 29% vs. n = 2, 4%; $p = 0.004$).

At week 52, additional resistance mutations to adefovir or entecavir were found in all patients with detectable HBV DNA whereas in 15% of patients in the adefovir plus lamivudine group ($p = 0.018$), and in none of the patients in the adefovir plus entecavir group. Safety and adverse event profiles were similar in the two groups. In conclusion, entecavir plus adefovir combination therapy provided superior virologic response and favorable resistance profiles, compared with continuing lamivudine plus adefovir combination, in patients with lamivudine-resistant HBV who fail to response to lamivudine plus adefovir combination therapy. [135] This combination is in phase IV clinical trial. [136]

2. Combination of Chemotherapeutic and Immunotherapeutic Agent(s)

A combination of chemotherapy and immunotherapy can result in regimens with enhanced therapeutic index with least side effects. In this combination, chemotherapy can bring down the viral load and at the same time immunotherapy can boost the innate and adaptive immune responses to clear the virus infected cells. This would also prove beneficial for reducing the instances of viral resistance associated with the long-term use of chemotherapeutic drugs alone and would reduce viral rebound after cessation of chemotherapy.

Lamivudine Plus Interferon

A review comprising nine controlled trials involving 942 patients has been reported for comparison of the effect and safety of lamivudine plus IFN-α combination therapy with lamivudine monotherapy, in patients with HBeAg-negative CHB. Among the trials, conventional interferon (CON-IFN) was used in eight trials (n=579) and PEG-IFN-α (n = 360), was used in one trial in combination with Lamivudine. Of these, two trials (n = 240) included antiviral treatment-naive patients, three studies (n=162) included IFN non-responders, and the remaining (n=540) included both IFN treatment-naive and previously treated patients.

In the review, the effect and safety of lamivudine monotherapy and its combination with IFN including CON-IFN and PEG-IFN for HBeAg-negative CHB patients was compared. No greater sustained virological and biochemical rates were observed in patients receiving CON-IFN/lamivudine combination therapy. However, combination group elicited a reduced YMDD mutation rate. No significant difference in the rate of treatment safety was observed between patients in the combination and monotherapy groups. No liver-related death was reported in the included trials. [137, 138]

Lamivudine Plus Peginterferon

This combination is discussed under the following headings.

Hepatitis B e Antigen–Positive Chronic Hepatitis

In a randomized and controlled trial, 307 patients with HBeAg-positive CHB were assigned to receive either the combination of lamivudine (100 mg/day) plus PEG IFN-α-2b (100 mg/week for 32 weeks, then 50 mg/week for 20 weeks), or PEG IFN-α-2b at the same dose plus placebo. At the end of the 26-week post-treatment follow-up, there was no difference in response rates between the two treatment groups. [139]

In another randomized, phase III study, 814 HBeAg-positive CHB patients received either PEG IFN-α-2a plus lamivudine (100 mg daily), PEG IFN-α-2a (180 mg once weekly) plus placebo, or lamivudine alone. Treatment was continued for 48 weeks and patients were followed up for an additional 24 weeks. The common adverse events were same as with therapies based on IFN-α. This study concluded that in HBeAg-positive CHB patients PEG-IFN-α-2a offers benefit over lamivudine, on the basis of HBeAg seroconversion, HBV DNA suppression, and HBsAg seroconversion. However no statistically significant differences in efficacy were found between the groups who received PEG-IFN-α-2a monotherapy and its combination with lamivudine after 24 weeks of follow-up. [140]

Hepatitis B e Antigen–Negative Chronic Hepatitis

In a phase III, partially double-blinded study the efficacy and the safety of PEG-IFN-α-2a alone or in combination with lamivudine versus lamivudine alone, was evaluated in 552 patients who were HBeAg-negative CHB. Patients were randomly assigned to receive 48 weeks of PEG IFN-α-2a (180 mg once weekly) plus lamivudine (100 mg once daily), PEG IFN-α-2a (180 mg once weekly) plus oral placebo (once daily), or lamivudine (100 mg once daily). This study revealed that in patients who have HBeAg-negative CHB, the efficacy of PEG IFN-α-2a monotherapy, as assessed 24 weeks after treatment, was superior to that of lamivudine monotherapy. The combination of PEG IFN-α-2a administered simultaneously with lamivudine was not superior to PEG IFN-α-2a used as monotherapy. [141] A 3-year follow-up data has been reported for a subgroup of patients (116/177 of those who received PEG IFN-α-2a plus placebo and 114/179 of those who received the PEG IFN plus lamivudine combination). Sustained off-therapy responses were maintained in about 30% of the patients who had HBeAg-negative CHB three years after treatment with PEG IFN-α-2a. In addition, loss of HBsAg was increased with time and was 8% at 3 years after treatment. [142, 143]

Telbivudine Plus Peginterferon

159 HBeAg-positive CHB patients were randomized to receive telbivudine (n = 55), PEG IFN (n=54), and PEG-IFN plus telbivudine (n=50). 110 patients reached treatment week 24, but the study was terminated early due to peripheral neuropathy (PN) events with PEG-IFN plus telbivudine. It was concluded that the combination of PEG-IFN plus telbivudine provided very potent antiviral efficacy with rapid and profound reduction in HBV DNA and HBsAg/HBeAg levels, but it carried an increased risk of PN. Despite increased efficacy, concomitant use of PEG-IFN and telbivudine should be avoided at present. [144] FDA has warned not to use this combination for HBV infections. [145]

Adefovir Plus Peginterferon

In a trial comprising of 57 HBeAg-positive CHB patients received PEGIFN-α-2a therapy for 48-week. At week 24, if serum HBV DNA levels exceeded 1000 copies/ml, the patients were assigned to group A (PEG-IFN-α2a plus adefovir, n = 21) or group B (PEG IFN-α-2a only, n = 14); otherwise, they were assigned to group C and received the constant monotherapy of PEG IFN-α-2a (n = 22). The results obtained in this study suggested that an adefovir add-on therapy in PEG-IFN-α-2a treatment might be able to improve the inhibition of HBV DNA in HBeAg positive CHB patients. However, a large, double-blind, randomized clinical trial is required to establish this observation. [146]

Phase IV study results of PEG-IFN-α-2a in combination with adefovir or entecavir in patients with HBeAg-positive CHB are awaited. [147]

Interleukin-12 (IL-12) Plus Lamivudine

Interleukin-12 (IL-12) is an immunomodulatory cytokine that promotes cellular immunity. Pre-clinical data suggest that IL-12 inhibits HBV replication by stimulating interferon-gamma (IFN-gamma) production. Several studies demonstrate that the treatment with lamivudine alone, or in combination with IL-12, result in the restoration of the HBV-specific CD4+ and CD8+ immune response in chronic HBV-infected individuals.

In a combination treatment study including lamivudine and recombinant human interleukin-12 (rhIL-12) versus lamivudine monotherapy, 15 patients with HBeAg-positive CHB were randomized to receive either lamivudine alone for 24 weeks (group 1); combination of lamivudine for 16 weeks and rhIL-12 (200 ng/kg twice weekly), starting 4 weeks after initiation of lamivudine, for 20 weeks (group 2), or the same schedule as for group 2, with lamivudine and a higher dose of rhIL-12 (500 ng/kg, group 3). Serum HBV DNA levels, T-cell proliferation, frequency of virus-specific T-cells, and IFN-gamma production were evaluated during and 24 weeks post-treatment. Lamivudine plus rhIL-12/500 showed higher antiviral activity than lamivudine monotherapy. However, after cessation of lamivudine treatment in groups 2 and 3, serum HBV DNA increased significantly despite continuing rhIL-12 treatment. Lamivudine plus rhIL-12 treatment showed greater increase in virus-specific T-cell reactivity and, IFN-gamma production. The report concluded that the addition of IL-12 to lamivudine enhances T-cell reactivity to HBV and IFN-gamma production. However, IL-12 does not abolish HBV replication in HBeAg-positive patients and does not maintain inhibition of HBV replication after lamivudine withdrawal. [148] The combination of IL-12 plus Lamivudine has not been explored much.

Conventional IFN Plus Ribavirin

A randomized study has been conducted on 119 patients to evaluate whether or not IFNα and ribavirin (**35**) combination therapy has a beneficial effect for HBeAg-positive CHB. 59 Patients received 5 million units of IFN-α2b daily for 4 weeks followed by 5 million units three times a week for 28 weeks, plus 1,200 mg ribavirin daily. 60 Patients received the same dosage of IFN plus placebo. The patients were followed for 24 weeks post-treatment, and 105 patients (88%) completed the entire course of 56 weeks. The results from this trial concluded that adding ribavirin does not increase the efficacy of IFN for the treatment of HBeAg-positive CHB. [149] Phase III trial including a randomized, multi-center, placebo-controlled study in patients with HBeAg-positive CHB has been completed. [150]

PEG- IFN Plus Ribavirin

In a randomized study, 138 HBeAg-negative CHB patients were included to receive monotherapy (PEG-IFNα-2a 180μg weekly plus placebo) or combination therapy (PEG-IFNα-α-2a weekly plus ribavirin 1,000 or 1,200mg daily, depending on body weight) for 48 weeks. Post-treatment follow-up was for 24 weeks. This combination therapy was well tolerated, although it was associated with a higher risk of anemia and neutropenia. Treatment with PEG-IFN-α-2a resulted in a limited sustained response rate in HBeAg-negative CHB patients and addition of ribavirin did not improve response to therapy. [151] This combination has completed phase III trial for patients with HBeAg negative chronic HBV infection. [152]

Thymosin Plus Lamivudine (Plus IFN)

Thymosins are small proteins present in various tissues in animals and have diverse biological functions. Thymosin-α-1 and β-4 have been utilized for therapy. In a study, 74 patients with HBeAg-positive CHB were categorized into sequential combination group (30 patients who received thymosin-α1 for 8 weeks, 6 months IFN treatment started in the 5th week, and lamivudine started 2 months later after HBeAg seroconversion or just after the stopping IFN, to more than 18 month), simultaneous combination group (14 patients who received 6 months IFN and thymosin-α1 simultaneously in the same manner as in sequential anti-viral group), and lamivudine group (30 patients who received lamivudine >18-month). HBeAg seroconversion, undetectable HBV DNA and normalization of ALT were found in 76.7%, 57.1% and 16.7% among the three groups, respectively ($p < 0.01$). Sequential anti-viral therapy had much higher rates of long-term efficacy. [153]

A randomized study has been conducted to elucidate whether the combination of Thymosin-α1 and lamivudine is superior to lamivudine monotherapy in HBeAg-positive naïve patients with CHB. 67 Patients were divided into groups as follows: the combination group (34 patients) received thymosin-α1 (1.6 mg, twice a week) and lamivudine (100 mg, daily) for 24 weeks, followed by continuous lamivudine therapy, the monotherapy group (n = 33) received lamivudine monotherapy continuously. No obvious benefit of virological and biochemical response was observed for combination treatment of thymosin-α1 and lamivudine as compared to the lamivudine monotherapy. In addition, after stopping thymosin-α1 treatment, the combination therapy was not effective to prevent viral and biochemical breakthroughs. [154]

However a database analysis of eight trials (total 583 patients) which was carried out to compare the effect of lamivudine monotherapy with that of lamivudine and thymosin α-1 combination therapy for the treatment of HBeAg-positive hepatitis B patients, suggested that the lamivudine and thymosin-α1 combination treatment was significantly superior to lamivudine treatment in terms of biochemical response ALT normalization rate, virological response rate, and HBeAg seroconversion rate. [155]

3. Combination Therapy Using Two Immunomodulators

Thymosin-α1 Plus IFN

A double-blinded, randomized, placebo-controlled trial was conducted for evaluation of therapeutic efficacy of IFN-α, and thymosin-α1 to determine if combination therapy was superior to IFN alone. The study compared the addition of thymosin-α1, 1.6 μg taken three times per week (combination therapy) or thymosin placebo (monotherapy) to lymphoblastoid IFN, 5 million international units (MIU) taken three times/week, for 24 weeks. Statistically no significant differences between the different therapies were found with respect to the secondary endpoints of HBeAg seroconversion, changes in histology, normalization of ALT or loss of HBV DNA. In conclusion, this trial showed a 17.8% improvement in HBeAg loss rates using combination therapy over IFN monotherapy. [156]

Vaccine Plus IFNs

In a randomized study, 50 treatment-naive children with CHB were assigned to receive either IFN-α-2b for 9 months, and pre-S2/S vaccine at the beginning and 4 and 24 weeks after initiation of IFN therapy (n = 25), or recombinant IFN-α-2b alone for 9 months (n = 25). At the end of the therapy, the mean HBV DNA values declined significantly in combination group

($p = 0.004$), but no statistically significant difference was found 6 months after the end of treatment [157].

Conclusion

Although current vaccine for Hepatitis B is very effective and has been used successfully worldwide for prophylaxis, the 350 million patients with CHB need effective and resistance free regimen(s). The present therapies include long duration treatment with no guarantee of complete viral clearance, and have fear of rebound after cessation of the therapy. The pipeline of hepatitis B drug development has potential chemo- and immunotherapeutic agents. We can envision that combination regimens would provide better clinical outcome, however, each combination, doses of drugs in combination, duration of treatment and toxicity profiles of drugs have to be seriously taken into account. Multiple clinical trials are underway but a successful treatment approach needs more intensive efforts and financial support. We, in near future, can hope finding better options to treat/cure this hepatic disease in reduced duration and with least complications.

References

[1] Barker, L. F, Shulman, N. R., Murray, R., Hirschman, R. J., Ratner, F., Diefenbach, W. C., Geller, H. M. Transmission of Serum Hepatitis. 1970. *Journal of the American Medical Association*, 1996, *276*, 841–844.

[2] Hunt, Richard (2007-11-21). *Hepatitis Viruses*. University of Southern California, Department of Pathology and Microbiology. Retrieved 2008-03-13.

[3] World Health Organization (WHO) *Fact Sheet 2008*; WHO Press: Geneva, Switzerland, 2008. Also see the website: http://www.who.int/mediacentre/factsheets/fs204/en/.

[4] Kennedy, M., Alexopoulos, S. P. Hepatitis B Virus Infection and Liver Transplantation. *Curr. Opin. Organ Transplant*. 2010, *15*, 310–315.

[5] Rapti, I. N., Hadziyannis, S. J. Treatment of Special Populations with Chronic Hepatitis B Infection. *Expert Review of Gastroenterology and Hepatology*. 2011, 5, (3), 323-339.

[6] Keating G. M., Noble S. Recombinant Hepatitis B Vaccine (Engerix-B): A Review of Its Immunogenicity and Protective Efficacy against Hepatitis B. *Drugs*. 2003, *63*, 1021-51.
[7] Bergman, S. J., Ferguson, M. C., Santanello, C. Biologic Response Modifiers in Infectious Disease *Infectious Disease Clinics of North America* 2011, *5*, 819-834.
[8] Ghany, M., Liang, T. J. Drug Targets and Molecular Mechanisms of Drug Resistance in Chronic Hepatitis B. *Gastroenterology*. 2007, *132*, 1574-1585.
[9] Kao, J.-H.; Chen, D. S. *Lancet Infect. Dis*. 2002, *2*, 395-403.
[10] Bock, C. T.; Schwinn, S.; Locarnini, S.; Fyfe, J.; Manns, M. P.; Trautwein, C.; Zentgraf, H. *J. Mol. Biol*. 2001, *307*, 183-196.
[11] Tacke, F.; Manns, M. P.; Trautwein, C. *Curr. Med. Chem*. 2004, *11*, 2667-2677.
[12] Delaney, W. E.; Locarnini, S.; Shaw, T. *Antiviral. Chem. Chemother*. 2001, *12*, 1-35.
[13] Deres, K.; Schroder, C. H.; Paessens, A.; Goldmann, S.; Hacker, H. J.; Weber, O.; Kramer, T.; Niewohner, U.; Pleiss, U.; Stoltefuss, J.; Graef, E.; Koletzki, D.; Masantschek, R. N. A.; Reimann, A.; Jaeger, R.; Grob, R.; Bekermann, B.; Schlemmer, K.- H.; Haebich, D.; Waigmann, H. R. *Science* 2003, *299*, 893-896.
[14] Lu, X.; Tran, T.; Simsek, E.; Block, T. M. *Journal of Virology*, 2003, *77*, 11933-11940.
[15] Kamiya, N.; Kubota, A.; Iwase, Y.; Sekiya, K.; Ubasawa, M.; Yuasa, S. *Antimicrob. Agents Chemother*. 2002, *46*, 2872-2877.
[16] Delaney IV, W. E.; Edwards, R.; Colledge, D.; Shaw, T.; Furman, P.; Painter, G.; Locarnini, S. *Antimicrob. Agents Chemother*. 2002, *46* , 3057-3060.
[17] King, R. W.; Ladner, S. K.; Miller, T. J.; Zaifert, K.; Perni, R. B.; Conway, S. C.; Otto, M. J. *Antimicrob. Agents Chemother*. 1998, *42*, 3179-3186.
[18] Rehermann, B. *Semin. Liver Dis*. 2003, *23* (Suppl. 1), 21.
[19] Lau, G. K.; Yiu, H. H.; Fong, D. Y. *Gastroenterology*, 2003, *125*, 1742-1749.
[20] (a) Idilman, R.; Arat, M.; Soydan, E. *J. Viral Hepat*. 2004, *11*, 141-147. (b) Urban, S.; Urban, S.; Fischer, K. P.; Tyrrell, D. L. *Proc. Natl. Acad. Sci. USA* 2001, *98*, 4984-4989.

[21] Nevens, F.; Main, J.; Honkoop, P.; Tyrrell, D. L.; Barber, J.; Sullivan, M. T.; Fevery, J.; De Man, R. A.; Thomas, H. C. *Gastroenterology* 1997, *113*, 1258-1263.

[22] Liaw, Y. F.; Leung, N. W.; Chang, T. T.; Guan, R.; Tai, D. I.; Ng, K. Y.; Chien, R. N.; Dent, J.; Roman, L.; Edmundson, S.; Lai, C. L. *Gastroenterology* 2000, *119*, 172-180.

[23] Yuen, M. F.; Sablon, E.; Hui, C. K.; Yuan, H. J.; Decraemer, H.; Lai, C. L. *Hepatology* 2001, *34*, 785-791.

[24] Sokal, E. *Exp. Opin. Pharmacother.* 2002, *3*, 329-339.

[25] Liaw, Y. F. *Antivir Chem Chemother* 2001, 12 (Suppl 1), 67-71.

[26] Papatheodoridis, G. V.; Dimou, E.; Dimakopoulos, K.; Manolakopoulos, S.; Rapti, I.; Kitis, G.; Tzourmakliotis, D.; Manesis, E.; Hadziyannis, S. J. *Hepatology*, 2005, *42*, 121-129.

[27] Zhang, Q. Q.; An, X; Liu, Y. H.; Li, S. Y.; Zhong, Q.; Wang, J.; Hu, H. D.; Zhang, D. Z.; Ren, H.; Hu, P.; *Virol. J.* 2011, *8*, 72.

[28] Heijtink, R. A.; De Wilde, G. A.; Kruining, J.; Berk, L.; Balzarini, J.; De Clercq, E.; Holy, A.; Schalm, S. W. *Antiviral Res.* 1993, *21*, 141-153.

[29] Perrillo, R.; Schiff, E.; Yoshida, E.; Statler, A.; Hirsch, K.; Wright, T.; Gutfreund, K.; Lamy, P.; Murray, A. *Hepatology*, 2000, *32*, 129-134.

[30] Gilson, R. J. C.; Chopra, K.; Murray, L. I. *Hepatology*, 1996, *24*, 281A.

[31] (a) Marcellin, P.; Chang, T. T.; Lim, S. G.; Tong, M. J.; Sievert, W.; Shiffman, M. L.; Jeffers, L.; Goodman, Z.; Wulfsohn, M. S.; Xiong, S.; Fry, J.; Brosgart, C. L. Adefovir Dipivoxil 437 Study Group. *Engl. J. Med.* 2003, *348*, 808-816; (b) Hadziyannis S. J.; Tassopoulos, N.; Heathcote, E. J.; Chang, T. T.; Kitis, G.; Rizzetto, M.; Marcellin, P.; Lim, S. G.; Goodman, Z.; Wulfsohn, M. S.; Xiong, S.; Fry, J.; Brosgart, C. L.; Adefovir Dipivoxil 438 Study Group. *Engl. J. Med.* 2003, *348*, 800-807.

[32] Hepsera prescribing information. Gilead Sciences Inc. 2002, 1-18.

[33] Marcellin, P.; Heathcote, E. J.; Buti, M. et al. *N. Engl. J. Med.* 2008, *359*, 2442-2455.

[34] Woo, G.; Tomlinson, G.; Nishikawa, Y. et al. *Gastroenterology*, 2010, *139*, 1218-1229.

[35] (a) Heathcote, E. J.; Gane, E.; DeMan, R. et al. (Abstract). *Hepatology*, 2007, *46* (Suppl 1), 861A; (b) Heathcote, E. J.; Marcellin, P.; Buti, M. et al. *Gastroenterology*, 2011, *140*, 132-143; (c) Snow-Lampart, A.; Chappell, B.; Curtis, M.; Zhu, Y.; Myrick, F.; Schawalder, J.; Kitrinos, K.; Svarovskaia, E. S.; Miller, M. D.; Sorbel, J.; Heathcote, J.; Marcellin, P.; Borroto-Esoda, K. *Hepatology*, 2011, *53*, 763-73.

[36] Herlitz, L. C.; Mohan, S.; Stokes, M. B. et al. *Kidney Int.* 2010, *78*, 1171-1177.

[37] Bryant, M. L.; Bridges, E. G.; Placidi, L.; Faraj, A.; Loi, A. G.; Pierra, C.; Dukhan D.; Gosselin, G.; Imbach, J. L.; Hernandez, B.; Juodawlkis, A. et al. *Nucleosides Nucleotides Nucleic Acids* 2001, *20*, 597-607.

[38] Bryant, M. L.; Bridges, E. G.; Placidi, L.; Faraj, A.; Loi, A. G.; Pierra,C.; Dukhan, D.; Gosselin, G.; Imbach, J. L.; Hernandez, B.; Juodawlkis, A et al. *Antimicrob. Agents Chemother.* 2001, *45*, 229-235.

[39] Keam S. J. *Drugs.* 2007, 67, 1917-1929.

[40] Hodge, R. A. *Curr. Opin. Investig. Drugs* 2004, *5*, 232-241.

[41] Bridges E. G. *J. Hepatol.*2006, *44* (Suppl 2): S147.

[42] Novirio Pharmaceuticals: Clinical Trial Update, *Genetic Engineering News* 2002, *22*, 59.

[43] Lai, C. L.; Gane, E.; Liaw, Y. F. et al. *N. Engl. J. Med.* 2007, *357*, 2576-2588.

[44] Locarnini S. *Hepatol Int* 2008, 2, 147-151.

[45] Seifer, M.; Hamatake, R. K.; Colonno, R. J.; Standring, D. N. *Antimicrob. Agents Chemother.* 1998, *42*, 3200.

[46] Baraclude (entecavir) prescribing information. Bristol-Myers Squibb Co. USA.

[47] Colonno, R.; Medina, I.; Lamb, C.; Genovesi, E.; Clark, J. *Hepatology*, 1998, *28*, 488A.

[48] (a) Lai, C. L.; Shouval, D.; Lok, A. S. et al. *N. Engl. J. Med.* 2006, *354*, 1011-1020;(b) Chang, T. T, Gish, R. G.; de Man, R. et al. *N. Engl. J. Med.* 2006, *354*, 1001-1010.

[49] (a) Tenney, D. J.; Rose, R. E.; Baldick, C. J. et al. *Hepatology* 2009, *49*, 1503-1514; (b) Kwak, M. S.; Choi, J. W.; Lee, J. S.; Kim, K. A.; Suh, J. H.; Cho, Y. S.; Won, S. Y.; Park, B. K.; Lee, C. K. *Journal of Viral Hepatitis* 2011, *18*, e432–e438; (c) Zhao, P.; Liu, W.; Zhao, J. and Q Guan. *Virology Journal* 2011, *8*, 75.

[50] (a) Ling, J. Y.; Zhang, G. Y.; Cui, Z. J.; Zhang, C. K. *J. Chromatogr., A* 2007, *1145*, 123–127.(b) Cai, X.; Wang, G. J.; Qu, Y.; Fan, C. H.; Zhang, R. Q; Xu, W. S. *Acad. J. Second Mil. Med. Univ.* 1997, *18*, 47–49.(c) Lu, L. G.; Zeng, M. D.; Mao, Y. M.; Li, J. Q.; Wan, M. B.; Li,C. Z.; Chen, C. W.; Fu, Q. C.; Wang, J. Y.; She, W. M.; Cai, X.; Ye,J.; Zhou, X. Q.; Wang, H.; Wu, S. M.; Tang, M. F.; Zhu, J. S.; Chen, W. X.; Zhang, H. Q. *J. Gastroenterol.* 2003, *9*, 2480–2483 (d) Wang, B. E. *Gastroenterol. Hepatol.* 2000, *15* (suppl. E), 67–70.

[51] (a) Gao L. M.; Han, Y. X.; Wang, Y. P.; Li, Y. H.; Shan, Y. Q.; Li, X.; Peng, Z. G.; Bi, C. W.; Zhang, T.; Du, N. N.; Jiang, J. D.; Song, D. Q. *J. Med. Chem.* 2011, *54*, 869–876.

[52] Zhang, L.; Wang, G.; Hou, W. Li P, Dulin, A.; Bonkovsky, H. L. *Hepatology* 2010, *51*, 690-698.

[53] Balakrishna, Pal S.; Liu, S. H.; Zhu, Y. L.; Chu, C. K.; Cheng, Y. C. *Antimicrob. Agents Chemother.* 1996, *40*, 380-386.

[54] Chu, C. K.; Boundinot, F. D.; Peek, S. F.; Hong, J. H.; Choi, Y.; Korba, B. E. et al. *Antiviral Therapy* 1998, *3* (Suppl. 3), 113.

[55] Aguesse-German, S.; Liu, S. H.; Chevallier, M.; Pichoud, C.; Jamard, C.; Borel, C.; Chu, C. K.; Trepo, C.; Cheng, Y. C.; Zoulim, F. *Antimicrob. Agents Chemother.* 1998, *42*, 369-376.

[56] Tennant, B.; Jacob, J.; Graham, L. A.; Peek, S.; Du, J.; Chu, C. K. *Antiviral Res.* 1997, *34*, A52 (Abs.).

[57] Zhu, Y.; Yamamoto, T.; Cullen, J.; Saputelli, J.; Aldrich, C. E.; Miller, D. S.; Litwin, S.; Furman, P. A.; Jilbert, A. R.; Mason, W. S. *J. Virol.* 2001, *75*, 311-322.

[58] Available from http://clinicaltrials.gov/ct2/show/NCT01264354?term= clevudineandrank=2 (Accessed in March 2012).

[59] De Clercq, E. *Int. J. Antimicrob. Agents* 1999, *12*, 81-95.

[60] Le Guerhier, F.; Pichoud, C.; Guerret, S.; Chevallier, M.; Jamard, C.; Hantz, O.; Li, X. Y.; Chen, S. H.; King, I.; Trepo, C.; Cheng, Y. C. et al. *Antimicrob. Agents Chemother.* 2000, *44*, 111-122.

[61] Le Guerhier, F.; Pichoud, C.; Jamard, C.; Guerret, S.; Chevallier, M.; Peyrol, S.; Hantz, O.; King, I.; Trepo, C.; Cheng, Y. C.; Zoulim, F. *Antimicrob. Agents Chemother.* 2001, *45*, 1065-1077.

[62] Dutschman, G. E.; Bridges, E. G.; Liu, S. H.; Gullen, E.; Guo, X.; Kukhanova, M.; Cheng, Y. C. *Antimicrob. Agents Chemother.* 1998, *42*, 1799-1804.

[63] Fu, L.; Cheng, Y. C. *Antimicrob. Agents Chemother.* 2000, *44*, 3402-3407.

[64] Ono, S. K.; Kato, N.; Shiratori, Y.; Kato, J.; Goto, T.; Schinazi, R. F.; Carrilho, F. J.; Omata, M. *J. Clin. Invest.* 2001, *107*, 449-455.

[65] Available from http://www.clinicaltrials.gov/ct2/show/NCT00034359? term=Elvucitabineandrank=8http://www.achillion.com/elvucitabine_data_overview (Accessed in March 2012).

[66] Chen, S. H. *Curr. Med. Chem.* 2002, *9*, 899-912.

[67] Furman, P. A.; Davis, M.; Liotta, D. C.; Paff, M.; Frick, L. W.; Nelson, D. J.; Dornsife, R. E.; Wurster, J. A.; Lawrence, J. W.; Fyfe, J. A.; Tuttle, J. V.; Miller, W. H.; Condreay, L.; Averett, D. R.; Schinazi, R. F.; Painter, G. R. *Antimicrob. Agents Chemother.* 1992, *36*, 2686-2692.

[68] Fourel, I.; Saputelli, J.; Schaffer, P.; Mason, W. S. *J. Virol.* 1994, *68*, 1059-1065.

[69] Korba, B. E.; Schinazi, R. F.; Cote, P.; Tennant, B. C.; Gerin, J. L. *Antimicrob. Agents Chemother.* 2000, *44*, 1757-1760.

[70] Cullen, J. M.; Smith, S. L.; Davis, M. G.; Dunn, S. E.; Botteron, C.; Cecchi, A.; Linsey, D.; Linzey, D.; Frick, L.; Paff, M. T.; Goulding, A et al. *Antimicrob. Agents Chemother.* 1997, *41*, 2076-2082.

[71] Gish, R.; Leung, N.; Wang. C.; Corey, L.; Sacks, S et al. *Am. Associa. Liver Dis.* 2002, Abs. 9838.

[72] Gish, R. G.; Leung, N. W. Y.; Wright, T. L. *Gastroenterology* 1999, *116A*, 1216.

[73] Dunkle, L. M. *ID Weekly Highlights* 2001, 30-32.

[74] Farrell G. C. *Drugs* 2000, *60*, 701-710.

[75] Das, K.; Xiong, X.; Yang, H.; Westland, C. E.; Gibbs, C. S.; Sarafianos, S. G.; Arnold, E. *J. Virol.* 2001, *75*, 4771-4779.

[76] Perrillo, R. P. *Seminars in Liver Disease* 2005, *25* (Suppl. 1), 20.

[77] Available from http://clinicaltrials.gov/ct2/results?term=emtricitabine+alone+hepatitis+b (Accessed in March 2012)

[78] Jacquard, A. C.; Brunelle, M. N.; Pichoud, C.; Durantel, D.; Carrouée-Durantel, S.; Trepo, C.; Zoulim, F. *Antimicrob Agents Chemother.* 2006, 50, 955-961.

[79] Schroder, I.; Holmgren, B.; Oberg, M.; Lofgren, B. *Antiviral Res.* 1998, *37*, 57-66.

[80] Lofgren, B.; Vickery, K.; Zhang, Y. Y.; Nordenfelt, E. *J. Viral Hepatitis* 1996, *3*, 61-65.

[81] Rajagopalan, P. F.; Boudinot, F. D.; Chu, C. K.; Mc-Clure, H. M.; Schinazi, R. F. *Pharm. Res.* 1994, *11* (suppl), 381.

[82] Chin, R.; Shaw, T.; Torresi, J.; Sozzi, V.; Trautwein, C.; Bock, T.; Manns, M.; Isom, H.; Furman, P.; Locarnini, S. *Antimicrob. Agents Chemother.* 2001, *45*, 2495-2501.

[83] Available from http://www.rfspharma.com/clinicalresearch.html.

[84] http://www.hepb.org/professionals/hbf_drug_watch.htm (Accessed in March 2012).

[85] Yuen, M. F.; Kim, J.; Kim, C. R.; Ngai, V.; Yuen, J. C.; Min, C.; Kang, H. M.; Shin, B. S.; Yoo, S. D.; Lai, C. L. *Antivir. Ther.* 2006, *11*, 977–983.
[86] Yuen, M. F.; Han, K. H.; Um, S. H.; Yoon, S. K.; Kim, H. R.; Kim, J.; Kim, C. R.; Lai, C. L. *Hepatology* 2010, *51*, 767–776.
[87] Reddy, K. R.; Matelich, M. C.; Ugarkar, B. G.;, Gómez-Galeno, J. E.; DaRe, J.; Ollis, K.; Sun, Z.; Craigo, W.; Colby, T. J.; Fujitaki, J. M.; Boyer, S. H.; van Poelje, P. D.; Erion, M. D. *J. Med. Chem.* 2008, *51*, 666-676.
[88] Available from http://clinicaltrials.gov/ct2/show/study/NCT00230503?term=Pradefovirandrank=1, (Accessed in March 2012).
[89] Srivastav, N. C.; Shakya, N.; Mak, M.; Agrawal, B.; Tyrrell, D. L.; Kumar R. *J. Med. Chem.* 2010, *53*, 7156–7166.
[90] Srivastav, N. C.; Shakya, N.; Mak, M.; Liang, C.; Tyrrell, D. L.; Agrawal, B.; Kumar, R. *Bioorg. Med. Chem.* 2010, *18*, 7542–7547.
[91] Kumar, R.; Tyrrell, D. L. *Bioorg. Med. Chem. Lett.* 2001, *11*, 2917-2920.
[92] Kumar, R.; Sharma, N.; Nath, M.; Saffran, H. A.; Tyrrell, D. L. *J. Med. Chem.* 2001, *44*, 4225-4229.
[93] Kumar, R.; Nath, M.; Tyrrell, D. L. *J Med. Chem.* 2002, *45*, 2032-2040.
[94] Semaine, W.; Johar, M.; Tyrrell, D. L. J.; Kumar, R.; Agrawal, B. *J. Med. Chem.* 2006, *49*, 2049-2054.
[95] Kumar, R.; Semaine, W.; Johar, M.; Tyrrell, D. L. J.; Agrawal, B. *J. Med. Chem.* 2006, *49*, 3693-3700.
[96] Perry, C. M.; Wagstaff, A. J. *Biodrugs*, 1998, *9*, 125-154.
[97] Maddrey, W. C. *Clin. Lab.* 2001, *47*, 51-55.
[98] Perrillo, R. P.; Schiff, E. R.; Davis, G. L.; Bodenheimer, H. C. Jr.; Lindsay, K.; Payne, J.; Dienstag, J. L.; O'Brien, C.; Tamburro, C.; Jacobson, I. M. *N. Eng. J. Med.* 1990, *323*, 295-301.
[99] Wong, D. K.; Cheung, A. M.; O'Rourke K.; Naylor, C. D.; Detsky, A. S.; Heathcote, *J. Ann. Intern. Med.* 1993, *119*, 312.
[100] Available from http://dailymed.nlm.nih.gov/dailymed/drugInfo.cfm?id=8326 (Accessed in March 2012).
[101] Pedder, S. C. *Semin. Liver Dis.* 2003, *23* (Suppl. 1), 19.
[102] Zeuzem, S.; Welsch, C.; Herrmann, E. *Semin. Liver Dis.* 2003, *23* (Suppl. 1), 23.
[103] Available from http://www.accessdata.fda.gov/drugsatfda_docs/label/2011/103964s5204lbl.pdf (Accessed in March 2012).
[104] Liu, C.- J.; Kao, J.- H. *Recent Pat. Anti-Infec. Drug Dis.* 2006, *1*, 85.

[105] Available from http://www.talecris-pi.info/inserts/hyperhepb.pdf (Accessed in March 2012).
[106] Available from http://www.fda.gov/downloads/BiologicsBloodVaccines/BloodBloodProducts/ApprovedProducts/LicensedProductsBLAs/FractionatedPlasmaProducts/ucm117658.pdf (Accessed in March 2012).
[107] Available from http://www.fda.gov/downloads/BiologicsBloodVaccines/BloodBloodProducts/ApprovedProducts/LicensedProductsBLAs/FractionatedPlasmaProducts/ucm119010.pdf (Accessed in March 2012).
[108] Available from http://clinicaltrials.gov/ct2/show/NCT00228592?term=Hepex-Bandrank=1 (Accessed in March 2012).
[109] (a) Available from http://www.replicor.com/debut_anglais2.htm (accessed in March 2012) (b) Al-Mahtab, M.; Bazinet, M.; Vaillant, A. Rep 9ac is a potent hbsag release inhibitor which clears serum hbsag and elicits svrs in patients with chronic hepatitis B,Oral Presentations, 01 APR, 2011, Available from http://www1.easl.eu/easl2011/program/Orals/339.htm (Accessed in March 2012).
[110] (a) Li, C.-L.; Zhang, T.; Saibara, T.; Nemoto, Y.; Ono, M.; Akisawa, N.; Iwasaki, S.; Maeda, T.; Onishi, S. *Int. Immunopharmacol.* 2002, *2*, 39-46. (b) Available from http://clinicaltrials.gov/ct2/show/NCT00291616?term=zadaxinandrank=7 (Accessed in March 2012).
[111] Lopatin, U.; Wolfgang, G.; Kimberlin, R. et al. A phase-I, randomized, double-blind, placebo-controlled study to evaluate the safety, tolerability, pharmacokinetics and pharmacodynamics of single escalating oral doses of GS-9620 in healthy subjects. 46th Annual Meeting of the European Association for the Study of the Liver (EASL 2011). Berlin. March 30-April 3. Available from http://www.hivandhepatitis.com/2011_conference/easl2011/docs/0412_2010_d.html (Accessed in March 2012).
[112] Available from http://www1.easl.eu/easl2011/program/Posters/Abstract628.htm (Accessed in March 2012).
[113] Available from http://www.dynavax.com/hepatitis_bt.html.
[114] Available from http://clinicaltrials.gov/ct2/show/NCT01023230 (Accessed in March 2012).
[115] Available from http://www.hbvadvocate.org/hepatitis/factsheets_pdf/HBV_Drugs_2008.pdf (Accessed in March 2012).
[116] (a) Urban, S.; Schulze, A.; Schieck, A.; Gähler, C.; Ni, Y.; Meier, A.; Alexandrov, A.; Mier W. *Journal of Hepatology* 2010, *52*, S5-S5.

[117] Lütgehetmann, M.; Mancke, L. V.; Volz, T.; Helbig, M.; Allweiss, L.; Bornscheuer, T.; Pollok, J. M.; Lohse, A. W.; Petersen, J.; Urban, S.; Dandri, M. *Hepatology*. 2012, *55*, 685-694.

[118] Available from http://www.cytheris.com/Pipeline/il7hbv.php, http:// www.cytheris.com/Clinical_Trials/hbv.php Accessed in March 2012).

[119] (a) Akbar, F. Sk. Md.; Horiike, N.; Onji, M. *World J. Gastroenterol.* 2006, *12*, 2876. (b) Farag, M. M.; Hoyler, B.; Encke, J.; Stremmel, W.; Weigand, K. *Vaccine*. 2010, *29*, 200-206.

[120] Yatsuji, H.; Suzuki, F.; Sezaki, H.; Akuta, N.; Suzuki, Y.; Kawamura, Y.; Hosaka, T.; Kobayashi, M.; Saitoh, S.; Arase, Y.; Ikeda, K.; Watahiki, S.; Iwasaki, S.; Kobayashi, M.; Kumada, H. *Journal of Hepatology,* 2008, *48*, 923–931.

[121] Chen, E.-Q.; Wang, L.-C.; Lei, J.; Xu, L.; Tang, H. *Virology Journal* 2009, 6, 163.

[122] Perrillo, R. P.; Hann, H. W.; Schiff, E.; Mutimer, D.; Willems, B.; Leung, N.; Lee, W. M.; Dixon, S.; Woessner, M.; Brosgart, C. L.; Condreay, L. D.; Gardner, S. D. *Hepatol. Int.* 2011, *5*, 654–663.

[123] Ghany, M. G.; Feld, J. J.; Zhao, X.; Heller, T.; Doo, E.; Rotman, Y.; Nagabhyru, P.; Koh, C.; Kleiner, D. E.; Wright, E. C.; Liang, T. J.; Hoofnagle, J. H. *Aliment Pharmacol. Ther.* 2012, in press.

[124] Available from http://clinicaltrials.gov/ct2/show/study/NCT01270165? term=LAMIVUDINE+PLUS+ADEFOVIR+DIPIVOXILandrank=1.

[125] Lai, C. L.; Leung, N.; Teo, E. K.; Tong, M.; Wong, F.; Hann, H. W.; Han, S.; Poynard, T.; Myers, M.; Chao, G.; Lloyd, D.; Brown, N. A. *Gastroenterology*. 2005, *129*, 528-536.

[126] Available from http://clinicaltrials.gov/ct2/show/NCT00275652?term= LAMIVUDINE+PLUS+TELBIVUDINEandrank=4 (Accessed in March 2012).

[127] Hui, C. K.; Zhang, H. Y.; Bowden, S.; Locarnini, S.; Luk, J. M.; Leung, K. W.; Yueng, Y. H.; Wong, A.; Rousseau, F.; Yuen, K. Y.; Naoumov, N. N.; Lau, G. K. *J. Hepatol.* 2008, *8*, 714-720.

[128] Liaw, Y. F.; Sheen, I. S.; Lee, C. M.; Akarca, U. S.; Papatheodoridis, G. V.; Suet-Hing Wong, F.; Chang, T. T.; Horban, A.; Wang, C.; Kwan, P.; Buti, M.; Prieto, M.; Berg, T.; Kitrinos, K.; Peschell, K.; Mondou, E.; Frederick, D.; Rousseau, F.; Schiff, E. R. *Hepatology* 2011, *53*, 62-72.

[129] Si-Ahmed, S. N.; Pradat, P.; Zoutendijk, R.; Buti, M.; Mallet, V.; Cruiziat, C.; Deterding, K.; Dumortier, J.; Bailly, F.; Esteban, R.; Wedemeyer, H.; Janssen, H. L.; Zoulim, F. *Antiviral Research* 2011, 92, 90–95.

[130] Available from http://clinicaltrials.gov/ct2/show/NCT00507507?term=TENOFOVIR+DISOPROXIL+PLUS+EMTRICITABINEandrank=1 (Accessed in March 2012).
[131] Petersen, J.; Ratziu, V.; Buti, M.; Janssen, H. L.; Brown, A.; Lampertico, P.; Schollmeyer, J.; Zoulim, F.; Wedemeyer, H.; Sterneck, M.; Berg, T.; Sarrazin, C.; Lutgehetmann, M.; Buggisch, P. *J. Hepatol.* 2012, *56*, 520-526.
[132] L. Milazzo, M. Corbellino, A. Foschi,V. Micheli, A. Dodero, A. Mazzocchi, V. Montefusco, G. Zehender,Antinori. S. *Transpl. Infect. Dis.* 2012, *14*, 95-98.
[133] Rago, A.; Lichtner, M.; Mecarocci, S.; Marocco, R.; Cenfra, N.; Belvisi, V.; Del, Borgo, C.; Cimino, G.; Mastroianni, C. M. *Antivir. Ther.* 2010, *15*, 929-932.
[134] Available fromhttp://clinicaltrials.gov/ct2/results?term=TENOFOVIR+DISOPROXIL+PLUS+ENTECAVIR (Accessed in March 2012).
[135] Lim, Y. S.; Lee, J. Y.; Lee, D.; Shim, J. H.; Lee, H. C.; Lee, Y. S.; Suh, D. J. *Antimicrob. Agents Chemother.* 2012, In press.
[136] Available from http://clinicaltrials.gov/ct2/show/NCT01023217?term=Adefovir+plus+Entecavirandrank=1 (Accessed in March 2012).
[137] Shi, Y.; Wu, Y. H.; Shu, Z. Y.; Zhang, W. J.; Yang, J.; Chen, Z. *HepatobiliaryPancreat Dis. Int.* 2010, *9*, 462-472.
[138] Available from http://clinicaltrials.gov/ct2/show/NCT00860626 (Accessed in March 2012).
[139] Janssen, H. L.; van Zonneveld, M.; Senturk, H.; Zeuzem, S.; Akarca, U. S.; Cakaloglu, Y.; Simon, C.; So, T. M.; Gerken, G.; de Man, R. A.; Niesters, H. G.; Zondervan, P.; Hansen, B.; Schalm, S. W. *Lancet* 2005, *365*, 123–129.
[140] Lau, G. K.; Piratvisuth, T.; Luo, K. X.; et al. *N. Engl. J. Med.* 2005, *352*, 2682–2695.
[141] Marcellin, P.; Lau, G. K.; Bonino, F. et al. *N. Engl. J. Med.* 2004, *351*, 1206–1217.
[142] (a) Asselah, T.; Lada, O.; Moucari, R.; Martinot, M.; Boyer, N.; Marcellin, P. *Clin. Liver Dis.* 2007, *11*, 839–849.
[143] Available from http://clinicaltrials.gov/ct2/show/NCT01095835?term=Lamivudine+plus+Peginterferonandrank=1 (Accessed in March 2012).
[144] Marcellin, P.; Avila, C.; Wursthorn, K.; Chuang, W.-L.; Lau, G. K.; Peng, C.-Y.; Gane, E. J.; Fainboim, H.; Manns, M. P.; Naoumov, N. V. *Journal of Hepatology* 2010, *52* | S1–S21.

[145] Available from www.hivandhepatitis.com/hepatitis-b/hepatitis-b-topics/hbv-treatment/533-hbv-drug-advisories-hbv-drug-advisories/3405-do-not-use-telbivudine-tyzeka-with-pegasys-for-hepatitis-b-fda-warns (Accessed in March 2012).

[146] Chen, L. B.; Shu, X.; Jie, Y. S.; Yang, X. A.; Zhang, K.; Li, G.; Xu, Q. H. *Zhonghua Shi Yan He Lin Chuang Bing Du XueZaZhi.*2010,*24*,39-41.

[147] http://www.roche-trials.com/studyResultGet.action?studyResultNumber=ML21827anddiseaseCategoryId=40.

[148] Rigopoulou, E. I.; Suri, D.; Chokshi, S.; Mullerova, I.; Rice, S.; Tedder, R. S.; Williams, R.; Naoumov, N. V. *Hepatology*. 2005, *42*, 1028-1036.

[149] Liu, C. J.; Lai, M. Y.; Chao, Y. C.; Liao, L. Y.; Yang, S. S.; Hsiao, T. J.; Hsieh, T. Y.; Lin, C. L.; Hu, J. T.; Chen, C. L.; Chen, P. J.; Kao, J. H.; Chen, D. S. *Hepatology*. 2006, *43*, 742-749.

[150] Available from http://clinicaltrials.gov/ct2/show/NCT00275938?term=IFN+Ribavirin+hepatitis+bandrank=2 (Accessed in March 2012).

[151] Rijckborst, V.; ter Borg, M. J.; Cakaloglu, Y.; Ferenci, P.; Tabak, F.; Akdogan, M.; Simon, K.; Raptopoulou-Gigi, M.; Ormeci, N.; Zondervan, P. E.; Verhey, E.; van Vuuren, A. J.; Hansen, B. E.; Janssen, H. L.; PARC Study Group A. *Am. J. Gastroenterol.* 2010, *105*, 1762–1769.

[152] Available from http://clinicaltrials.gov/ct2/results?term=PEG-+IFN+plus+Ribavirin (Accessed in March 2012).

[153] Available from http://www.medscape.com/viewarticle/578682_9 (Accessed in March 2012).

[154] Lee, H. W.; Lee, J. I.; Um, S. H.; Ahn, S. H.; Chang, H. Y.; Park, Y. K.; Hong, S. P.; Moon, Y. M.; Han, K. H. *J. Gastroenterol. Hepatol.* 2008, *23*, 729-735.

[155] Zhang, Y. Y.; Chen, E. Q.; Yang, J.; Duan, Y. R.; Tang, H. *Virology Journal* 2009, *6*, 63.

[156] Lim, S. G.; Wai, C. T.; Lee, Y. M.; Dan, Y. Y.; Sutedja, D. S.; Wee, A.; Suresh, S.; Wu, Y. J.; Machin, D.; Lim, C. C.; Fock, K. M.; Koay, E.; Bowden, S.; Locarnini, S.; Ishaque, S. M. *Antivir. Ther.* 2006, 11, 245-253.

[157] Helvaci, M.; Kizilgunesler, A.; Kasirga, E.; Ozbal, E.; Kuzu, M.; Sozen, G. *J. Gastroenterol. Hepatol.* 2004, *19*, 785-791.

In: Hepatitis B: New Research
Editors: J. T. Cox and D. I. Owen
ISBN 978-1-62081-846-6

Chapter II

Hepatitis B and Dialysis

Bhadran Bose[1], Katherine A. Barraclough[1], E. Geoffrey Playford[2] and David W. Johnson[1]*

[1]Department of Nephrology,
Princess Alexandra Hospital, Brisbane, Australia
[2]Infection Management Services,
Princess Alexandra Hospital, Brisbane, Australia

Abstract

There has been a substantial decrease in the incidence of hepatitis B virus (HBV) infection among dialysis populations, largely due to improvements in infection control procedures and the widespread implementation of HBV vaccination.

However dialysis patients remain at increased risk of HBV infection acquisition because of their increased exposure to blood products, shared dialysis equipment, frequent breaches of skin, and immunodeficiency. The rate of serum hepatitis B surface antigen (HBsAg) seropositivity in patients on maintenance haemodialysis in the developed world is low; although sporadic outbreaks of acute HBV infection continue to occur in

* Address for Correspondence: Professor David Johnson, Department of Nephrology, Level 2, ARTS Building, Princess Alexandra Hospital, Ipswich Road, Woolloongabba, Brisbane Qld 4102, AUSTRALIA, Tel: +61 7 3176 5080, Fax: +61 7 3176 5480, Email: david_johnson@health.qld.gov.au

this setting. The natural history of HBV among patients undergoing long-term dialysis remains unclear.

HBV-related liver disease is frequently asymptomatic in dialysis patients and liver-related mortality in this population is very low. There are no rigorously controlled trials for treatment of hepatitis B with either interferon or lamivudine therapy in dialysis patients currently available.

This chapter reviews the epidemiology, modes of transmission, diagnosis, prevention and treatment of HBV. Strategies to improve vaccination response, new therapeutic options and selection of patients for therapy will be specifically discussed.

Introduction

Hepatitis B Virus (HBV) is a major global health problem. More than one-third of the world's population is estimated to have been infected with HBV, and the World Health Organisation estimates that HBV results in 1 – 2 million deaths every year. HBV is highly infectious compared to other blood-borne viruses. An untreated percutaneous exposure to an infected source carries a risk of seroconversion of up to 30%, depending upon the degree of viraemia. By contrast, the risk of Hepatitis C virus and Human Immunodeficiency virus are 1.8% and 0.3% respectively [1].

Persistent carriage of HBV, defined by the presence of Hepatitis B surface antigen (HBsAg) in the serum for more than six months, has been estimated to affect about 350 million people worldwide [2].

The pathology is mediated by the host cellular immune response to the infected hepatocytes. Long term, continuing viral replication may lead to progressive chronic liver disease, cirrhosis and hepatocellular carcinoma.

Compared to the general population, dialysis patients are at increased risk of acquiring HBV.

Reasons include increased exposure to blood products, shared haemodialysis equipment, skin breaches, and immunodeficiency. Haemodialysis (HD), which requires access to the bloodstream, also affords an opportunity for transmission of HBV between patients, and between patients and staff. Viral hepatitis complicating haemodialysis has been recognized from the earliest days of this therapy.

While the introduction of vaccination programs and stringent infection control measures have succeeded in limiting the spread of hepatitis infection within dialysis facilities, outbreaks continue to occur periodically and prevalence rates remain unacceptably high. As such, HBV infection remains an important issue in renal replacement therapy.

Epidemiology

Hepatitis B occurs in people of all age groups with approximately the same incidence throughout the year. Transmission may occur vertically or horizontally through percutaneous and/or mucosal exposure to infected blood or body fluids [3]. More than 75% of the people in world with chronic hepatitis B infection live in the Asia-Pacific region; other highly endemic regions include Africa and the Amazon basin. Among such regions, the cumulative lifetime infection rate is above 50%, with more than 8% of the population being chronic carriers [4]. Infection in such regions is typically acquired in childhood, either horizontally from other children, or vertically from maternal carriers. By contrast, vertical transmission is rare in Australia, with parenteral transmission predominating, and fewer than 2% of the population being chronic HBV carriers.

The wide range in HBV carrier rates in different parts of the world is largely related to differences in the age at infection, which is inversely related to the risk of chronicity. The rate of progression from acute to chronic HBV infection is approximately 90% for perinatally-acquired infection (5), 20 to 50% for infections acquired between the ages of 1- 5, and less than 5% for adult-acquired infection [6, 7].

Hepatocellular carcinoma is the 6th most common cancer worldwide, and half of all cases are caused by HBV [8].

Historically, HBV has been a critical infection issue with haemodialysis facilities [9, 10]. Considerable transmission of HBV can occur between haemodialysis patients and staff [11]. Haemodialysis patients are at increased risk for HBV infection because of the opportunity for exposure to HBV associated with the dialysis procedure. The reservoir of infection for potential transmission of HBV is greater in haemodialysis patients. After infection with HBV, haemodialysis patients are at greater risk of becoming chronic carriers than the general population [11-13]. Moreover, the seroconversion rate after vaccination is less for chronic haemodialysis patients than for the general population (50-80% vs. >95%) [14-17]. The impaired immune response is presumed to be caused by uraemia-induced defects in phagocytosis and T- and B-cell function [18, 19]. Although many patients with end-stage renal disease

(ESRD) do not live long enough to develop HBV-related complications, there are reports of increased risks of hepatocellular carcinoma and mortality associated with HBV in the ESRD population [20, 21]. HBV infection is also associated with greater morbidity and mortality in ESRD patients after they have received a renal transplant [22-25].

Before the advent of vaccination, some success in limiting the spread of HBV was achieved by dialysing seropositive patients separately from those who were seronegative. This followed the 1972 publication of the Rosenheim Report in the United Kingdom (26). The report set out a code of practice for reducing transmission of hepatitis amongst dialysis patients. In 1977, guidelines were published in the U.S. to reduce HBV infection in dialysis units [27].

The incidence of new hepatitis B infections in US dialysis patients subsequently fell from 6.2% in 1974 to 1% by 1980 (28). Testing of a vaccine began in the 1970s, and this came into widespread clinical use from the early 1980s (29, 30). This further reduced the risk of HBV infection in the dialysis setting. Nevertheless, although rates of new infection are now low (31), hepatitis B continues to exist in dialysis populations. Prevalence rates tend to be dependent on baseline population rates. An analysis of data from the Dialysis Outcomes and Practice Patterns Study (DOPPS) showed a HBV prevalence of 0% - 6.6% across dialysis facilities in Western Europe, Japan and the US [32]. In contrast, a registry study of Asia-Pacific countries found the prevalence of HBsAg positivity ranged between 1.3-14.6% [33]. Reports from much smaller cohorts elsewhere have indicated HBsAg positivity rates of 13.3% in Turkey and 2.4% - 10% in Brazil [34-36].

HBV Transmission within Dialysis Units

Patients with chronic kidney disease (CKD) have impaired host defences against viral infections [37]. Consequently, the risk of acquisition is increased in dialysis populations regardless of dialysis modality. Prior to the introduction of erythropoietin therapy, CKD patients were also at increased risk of infection via transfusion of contaminated blood products.

The haemodialysis procedure presents an opportunity for blood contact with contaminated equipment, injection of liquids harboring virus, and exposure of breached skin or mucous membranes to infection. HBV is particularly able to persist with retained infectivity within the inanimate environment (38). Moreover, dialysis patients are more likely to be hospitalized and to require interventional procedures or surgery [39].

Historically, groups of patients in early peritoneal dialysis (PD) programmes were dialysed in-centre using intermittent PD. Because PD effluent from HBsAg positive patients is potentially infectious [40], this regular gathering of patients facilitated transmission of HBV. As a consequence, early infection risks were similar for PD and HD [41]. With the development of PD as a predominantly home therapy, rates of HBV infection in this population have fallen, so that the prevalence of HBV in PD populations is now heavily influenced by the underlying population prevalence. In countries with very high HBV endemicity, both PD and HD programmes have similar rates of seropositivity, reflecting HBV acquired before the commencement of dialysis [42, 43]. Conversely, in countries with low background prevalence, present-day risk of HBV in PD patients is associated with exposure to blood products and previous time spent on haemodialysis.

Most countries have guidelines for HBV infection control in dialysis units. All these guidelines underpin established infection control principles. These include vaccination, screening of haemodialysis patients, segregation/cohorting of potentially infectious patients, appropriate management of sharps, and avoidance of multi-dose vials for parenteral drugs. Other developments that have contributed to a reduction in infection risk include a widespread move from reusable membranes towards disposable dialysers and the introduction of synthetic erythropoietin with a decrease in the requirements for blood transfusion.

Dialysis unit staff members are also at increased risk of infection through exposure during the dialysis procedure. Infection with HBV compromises their own health, and risks further staff-to-patient transmission of HBV. Vaccination of all dialysis unit staff is recommended by guidelines, and response rates are >90% [44]. Non-responders who are HBsAg positive should be counseled and assessed accordingly and those who are HBsAg negative should be warned to seek post-exposure prophylaxis in the event of contact with potentially infectious blood. Other steps that can be taken to prevent cross infection with HBV between patients and staff include barrier protection, such as wearing gloves and face shields. Cleaning hands and changing gloves between contacts prevents staff infecting one patient from another. Minimising staff turnover and allocating dedicated staff to infectious patients is important. Full guidelines relating to management of occupational exposure to HBV, including percutaneous injuries, is available from the Centers for Disease Control (http://www.cdc.gov/mmwr/preview/mmwrhtml/rr5011a1.htm).

Despite the successes of these measures, HBV outbreaks continue to occur sporadically in haemodialysis units. These do not point to inadequacies in infection control guidelines, but rather to shortcomings in following such recommendations. In a review of 30 nosocomial HBV outbreaks since 1992, ten occurred in a haemodialysis setting [45]. The most common transmission pathways for these infections were multi-use drug vials (30.3%) and non-disposable capillary blood sampling devices (27.3%). An analysis of five HBV outbreaks in the U.S. during 1994 found that patients were infected through failures of isolation, serological screening and vaccination and through sharing of staff, equipment and supplies between patients [46].

Hepatitis B Serologic Markers

Infection with HBV is associated with characteristic changes in the serum levels of hepatitis B antigens and antibodies. These markers are used to define different clinical states.

Hepatitis B Surface Antigen and Antibody

HBsAg is the serologic hallmark of HBV infection. It can be detected by radioimmunoassays (RIA) or enzyme immunoassays (EIA).

HBsAg appears in serum 1-10 weeks after an acute exposure to HBV, prior to the onset of hepatitic symptoms or elevation of serum alanine aminotransferase (ALT).

In patients who subsequently recover, HBsAg usually becomes undetectable after four to six months. Persistence of HBsAg for more than six months implies chronic infection. It is estimated that less than 1 percent of immunocompetent adult patients with genuine acute hepatitis B progress to chronic infection [47]. Among patients with chronic HBV infection, the rate of clearance of HBsAg is approximately 0.5 percent per year [48].

The disappearance of HBsAg is followed by the appearance of hepatitis B surface antibody (anti-HBs). In most patients, anti-HBs persists for life, thereby conferring long-term immunity. In some patients, however, anti-HBs may not be detectable until after a window period of several weeks to months, during which neither HBsAg nor anti-HBs can be detected. At this time, the serologic diagnosis may be made by the detection of IgM antibodies against hepatitis B core antigen (IgM anti-HBc).

HBV can be classified into seven genotypes and four major serotypes. All HBV serotypes share one common antigenic determinant: "a." These serotypes have epidemiologic significance. Antibodies to the "a" determinant confer protection to all HBV serotypes [49].

Coexistence of HBsAg and anti-HBs has been reported in approximately 24 percent of HBsAg positive individuals [50]. In most instances, the antibodies are unable to neutralize the circulating virions. These individuals should therefore be regarded as carriers of the hepatitis B virus.

Hepatitis B Core Antigen and Antibody

Hepatitis B core antigen (HBcAg) is an intracellular antigen that is expressed in infected hepatocytes. It is not detectable in serum. Anti-HBc can be detected throughout the course of HBV infection.

During acute infection, anti-HBc is predominantly of IgM class. IgM anti-HBc is the sole marker of HBV infection during the window period between the disappearance of HBsAg and the appearance of anti-HBs. The detection of IgM anti-HBc is usually regarded as an indication of acute HBV infection.

However, IgM anti-HBc may remain detectable up to two years after the acute infection. Furthermore, the titer of IgM anti-HBc may increase to detectable levels during exacerbations of chronic hepatitis B [51]. This can present a diagnostic problem, incorrectly suggesting acute hepatitis B, particularly in endemic areas in which many HBsAg-positive patients presenting with acute hepatitis actually have exacerbations of chronic hepatitis B [7, 47]. Other common causes of acute exacerbation of chronic hepatitis B are superinfection with hepatitis D virus (delta virus) or hepatitis C virus [7, 47]. IgG anti-HBc persists along with anti-HBs in patients who recover from acute hepatitis. It also persists in association with HBsAg in those who progress to chronic HBV infection.

Isolated Anti-HBc

The isolated presence of anti-HBc in the absence of HBsAg and anti-HBs has been reported in 0.4 to 1.7 percent of blood donors in low prevalence areas and in 10 to 20 percent of the population in endemic countries [52]. Isolated detection of anti-HBc can occur in three settings: during the window period of acute hepatitis B when the anti-HBc is predominantly IgM class; many years after recovery from acute hepatitis B when anti-HBs has fallen to undetectable levels; and after many years of chronic HBV infection when the HBsAg titer has decreased below the cutoff level for detection. As noted above, loss of detectable HBsAg occurs in approximately 0.5 percent of patients with chronic hepatitis B per year [48].

The clinical significance of isolated anti-HBc is unclear. Although HBV DNA has been detected in the serum of individuals with isolated anti-HBc when tested by PCR assays, the frequency of detection varies from 0 to 20 percent [53]. HBV DNA can be detected in the liver of most (more than 70 percent) persons with isolated anti-HBc. Transmission of HBV infection has been reported from blood and organ donors with isolated anti-HBc but the incidence ranged widely from 0.4 to 78 percent [53-55]. The risk is highest when livers from anti-HBc positive donors are transplanted.

Studies in the late 1980s suggest that (based upon the development of a primary anti-HBs response to hepatitis B vaccination of asymptomatic individuals with isolated anti-HBc) as many as 50-80% of persons with isolated anti-HBc have false positive test results [52, 56]. Nonspecific results appear to be more common with anti-HBc enzyme immunoassays than with radioimmunoassays. However, improvement of enzyme immunoassays in the past decade has decreased the rate of false positive results.

The evaluation of individuals with isolated anti-HBc should include repeat testing for anti-HBc, HBsAg, anti-HBe, and anti-HBs. Those who remain isolated anti-HBc positive should be tested for the presence of IgM anti-HBc to rule out recent HBV infection. The presence of anti-HBe indicates that the individual had prior exposure to HBV. Individuals with evidence of chronic liver disease should be tested for HBV DNA to exclude low level chronic HBV infection.

Hepatitis B E Antigen and Antibody

Hepatitis B e antigen (HBeAg) is a secretory protein that is processed from the precore protein. It is generally considered to be a marker of HBV replication and infectivity. The presence of HBeAg is usually associated with high levels of HBV DNA in serum and higher rates of transmission of HBV infection from carrier mothers to their babies [57, 58] and from patients to health care workers [59].

HBeAg to anti-HBe seroconversion occurs early in patients with acute infection, prior to HBsAg to anti-HBs seroconversion. However, HBeAg seroconversion may be delayed for years to decades in patients with chronic HBV infection. In such patients, the presence of HBeAg is usually associated with the detection of high levels of HBV DNA in serum and active liver disease. However, HBeAg-positive patients with perinatally acquired HBV infection may have normal serum ALT concentrations and minimal inflammation in the liver [60].

Seroconversion from HBeAg to anti-HBe is usually associated with a decrease in serum HBV DNA and remission of liver disease [61, 62]. However, some patients continue to have active liver disease after HBeAg seroconversion [63, 64]. Such individuals may have low levels of wild type HBV or HBV variants with a stop codon in the precore or dual nucleotide substitutions in the core promoter region that prevent or decrease the production of HBeAg [65].

Hepatitis B Vaccination

The Hepatitis B Vaccine

In the 1970s, Krugman observed that HBsAg was immunogenic, and that anti-HBs antibodies were protective against hepatitis B [66]. A first-generation vaccine was subsequently developed, consisting of HBsAg extracted by plasmapheresis from HBV carriers, and then inactivated [67]. This vaccine, manufactured by Merck, was approved by the FDA in 1981, and became widely available from July 1982. A similar vaccine was licensed at about the same time, produced by Institut Pasteur in France.

Modern "second generation" HBV vaccines are recombinant non-infectious subunit vaccines containing HBsAg [68]. These are produced by the yeast Saccharomyces cerevisiae using recombinant DNA technology. There are two such HBV vaccine formulations available, Engerix B and Recombivax HB.

A third-generation vaccine has been produced from a mammalian cell line, although it is not yet in widespread use. It contains the pre-S1 and pre-S2 antigens that are present on the viral envelope. These antigens are more immunogenic than the HBsAg present in second-generation vaccines [69].

Whichever vaccine is used, providing manufacturer's recommendations are adhered to, immunogenicity and efficacy are considered equivalent [70]. In line with Krugman's earlier observations, efficacy studies have shown that at least 90% of subjects developing anti-HBs levels of 10 IU/L are protected from hepatitis B infection [71]. Safety data are comprehensive. A large prospective trial has shown the vaccine to be safe and well tolerated [72].

Efficacy of Hepatitis B Vaccine

Szmuness et al demonstrated the efficacy of the first-generation, plasma-derived HBV vaccine (PDV) in 1980 in a randomized, double-blind placebo-controlled trial (RCT) in a high-risk population with normal renal function [73]. The same group then investigated use of the Merck vaccine in 79 U.S. haemodialysis patients and demonstrated that 89% produced detectable anti-HBs [30].

The Pasteur vaccine was examined in an RCT of 138 dialysis patients. Despite a low seroconversion rate of 60%, the vaccine was protective when compared to placebo (74). Another observational study of the Merck vaccine found seroconversion rates of 50% in male HD patients and 66% in females. By contrast, 100% of 7 predialysis patients had protective antibody [17]. Szmuness' group reported the largest RCT of HD patients in 1984 (n=1311) [75]. A three-dose schedule produced a 50% response rate. Two other early studies found seroconversion rates in HD patients of 60-75% (29, 76). The second of these, a Dutch RCT, replicated the findings of the prior French study [77], showing that the vaccine was protective against HBV infection compared to placebo. The overall message from all these trials of HBV vaccine in haemodialysis patients was that HD patients were substantially less responsive to the vaccine than healthy individuals, but that the vaccine did confer protection from HBV infection. There was a suggestion that women responded better than men to vaccination. The second-generation or yeast-derived vaccine (YDV) was found to have similar efficacy in healthy recipients to the earlier PDV. An early investigation found 97% seroconversion in 32 HD patients with the YDV [78]. Bruguera et al examined the YDV in over 270 HD patients [15]. Using a four-dose schedule and dosing at 0, 1, 2 and 6 months with 40 μg vaccine, 69% of patients achieved an anti-HBs titre of ≥10 IU/L (considered protective). If the fourth dose was given at 12 months, the seroprotection rate reached 76%.

Strategies for Improving Immune Response

When the vaccine is used in immune-competent individuals using a three-dose schedule, a 90%-95% seroprotection rate is expected. Clearly, in vaccine recipients with renal failure, the rates are substantially lower. In an attempt to improve seroconversion rates, current recommendations state that dialysis patients should receive higher vaccine doses than individuals with normal renal function. As such, 40 µg of Recombivax HB at 0, 1 and 6 months, or 40µg of Engerix-B at 0, 1, 2 and 6 months should be administered. The best reported response rates to these schedules are <85% achieving seroprotection [79, 80].

Not only is the response to the vaccine blunted, but anti-HBs levels decline more rapidly after immunization in haemodialysis patients compared with healthy individuals, such that in 41% of responsive patients the levels are undetectable at three years [81]. Other reports suggest that in up to 42% there are no detectable anti-HBs levels one year after vaccination.

The likelihood of a seroconversion response to hepatitis B vaccine decreases as renal failure progresses. As mentioned above, Köhler et al found a far superior response to the PDV in their small group of predialysis patients [17]. This has been borne out by other studies more recently using YDV [82, 83]. As a result, guidelines also recommended that patients with CKD be vaccinated as early as possible in the course of their renal disease. Although vaccinating patients prior to dialysis makes immunological sense, there are substantial cost implications in vaccinating much larger numbers of patients: Many predialysis patients will never progress to renal replacement therapy, succumbing instead to their comorbidities.

Vaccine adjuvants have been studied in HD patients. The addition of granulocyte-macrophage colony-stimulating factor and interleukin-2 has not been consistently successful in improving response rates [84, 85]. Likewise, studies have failed to show a significant, durable benefit of interferons or thymopentin [86-88].

Alternatively, a more recent vaccine formulation (HBV-AS04) consisting of standard Engerix-B YDV with adjuvant 3-O-desacyl-40-monophosphoryl lipid A, has shown the ability to provide earlier and greater anti-HBs responses than the standard vaccine [89]. More importantly, a small follow-up study has shown that the rate of decline in seroprotectivity was slower for the HBV-AS04 vaccine [90]. As such, this is the most promising vaccine adjuvant to date. It was licensed for use in CKD patients in Europe in 2005.

Finally, studies have investigated whether intradermal (ID) vaccination may afford improved seroconversion. HBV vaccination in healthcare workers was evaluated in a Cochrane review in 2005 [91]. Low-dose intradermal injection was shown to provide lower anti-HBs levels than high-dose intramuscular vaccination in this immunocompetent group of recipients. The following year a meta-analysis of IM versus ID vaccination in haemodialysis patients concluded that the intradermal route generated a superior anti-HBs response at the end of the vaccination protocol, but no significant differences in antibody levels were seen over longer follow-up [92].

A similar conclusion was reached from a single, small study of 60 CAPD patients who were randomized to ID or IM vaccination [93]. The peak anti-HBs titres were reached earlier in the ID group, and a higher seroconversion rate attained, but there was no difference between the two groups in maintenance of seroprotective anti-HBs levels over 2 years of follow-up.

The intradermal route is more technically challenging and causes an increased incidence of local reactions. Given that the majority of dialysis patients will respond to primary IM vaccination, the deltoid intramuscular route seems preferable for primary vaccination, with the ID route reserved for the more troublesome group of non-responders.

The antibody response to Hepatitis B vaccination declines with time. It is current practice to administer booster doses to those with an adequate initial response whose anti-HBs levels fall below 10 IU/l.

For those who do not respond adequately to the initial vaccination course, a re-vaccination schedule may be employed. Bock et al assessed the effect of a shorter re-vaccination course of injections in a small group of haemodialysis patients [94]. In this randomized controlled trial, no improved efficacy for a shorter re-vaccination schedule was demonstrated.

By contrast Barraclough et al used 8 weekly ID injections of low-dose HBV vaccine in patients initially unresponsive to a standard vaccination schedule [95]. In a randomized comparison with a 2-dose, 8-week IM vaccination schedule, the patients receiving ID vaccination had a significantly greater seroconversion rate, with a trend towards longer seroprotection in responders.

The ID injections were well-tolerated. The findings were consistent with a prospective, randomized study from Italy in 1997 [96]. Alternatively, a small observational study from Israel found that the use of the third-generation vaccine Bio-Hep-B in a revaccination protocol yielded seroprotective anti-HBs levels in 25 of 29 initial non-responders (86%) to a standard vaccination schedule [97].

Patients should therefore be vaccinated according to guidelines, with the recommended "double dose" of 40μg. If there is no response a second series can be given. If the initial response is adequate, but anti-HBs levels fall to <10IU/l, a booster dose should be given. Those who do not produce protective levels (≥10IU/l) of anti-HBs after 2 series might be considered for ID vaccination, or the third-generation vaccine.

Treatment of Hepatitis B in Dialysis Patients

Dialysis patients with chronic HBV infection should have regular monitoring of parenchymal and ductal liver enzymes, and serum albumin concentration, preferably at six to eight week intervals. Prothrombin time should also be measured when there is evidence of severe hepatitis or cirrhosis. In addition, serum alpha-fetoprotein levels should be measured every three to four months and liver ultrasound performed at least annually.

Since the biochemical manifestations often cannot reliably indicate the status of liver histology, it would be ideal if a liver biopsy is available to best assess the activity of HBV related liver disease and the extent of cirrhotic changes [98, 99].

However, the role and optimal timing of liver biopsy in otherwise asymptomatic patients without clinical or biochemical abnormalities remain to be defined. Decisions on management for an individual patient must also take into consideration the level of HBV DNA in serum and the estimated waiting time before a kidney allograft is available.

Liver biopsy is recommended when anti-viral treatment is being considered. Availability of histological information is also preferred before kidney transplantation, to ascertain the activity of hepatitis and the degree of cirrhosis. However, while it is easy to arrange liver biopsy before living-donor kidney transplantation, the optimal timing for this procedure may be difficult to establish in localities with a long waiting time for transplantation.

Decisions on the treatment of chronic HBV infection are based in part upon an accurate assessment of the presence or absence of virus replication and active liver disease [100]. This usually involves testing for HBV DNA and

HBeAg, measuring the serum ALT concentration, with or without a liver biopsy.

Treatment is often indicated when abnormal ALT levels suggest evidence of hepatic inflammation and HBV DNA levels are 4 to 5 log10 copies/mL or above. Based upon these and other clinical findings, optimal therapy may involve the administration of interferon-alfa, nucleoside or nucleotide analogues, combination therapy, liver transplantation, or only observation.

A paucity of data exists concerning the optimal therapy of chronic HBV infection in dialysis patients. A few small studies have examined the use of interferon-alfa and nucleoside or nucleotide analogues in this patient population.

Interferon-Alfa

There are little data on interferon-alfa treatment in dialysis patients with HBV infection. Improvement in liver biochemistry and HBe seroconversion was observed in two patients after treatment with 3 MU of interferon-alfa thrice weekly for three months, with follow-up durations of nine months and four years, respectively [101].

In contrast to patients without renal failure, in whom interferon-alfa therapy is generally well tolerated, the side effects of standard interferon-alfa are more pronounced in dialysis patients, especially with regard to the exacerbation of anemia and protein malnutrition [102, 103]. Preliminary data suggest that pegylated interferon might be better tolerated in patients with renal failure, although its efficacy and safety in hepatitis B treatment in this patient population remains undefined [104].

Nucleoside or Nucleotide Analogues

Lamivudine is an oral nucleoside analogue that interferes with the reverse transcriptase of HBV and terminates the nascent proviral DNA. It is the first in this class of drugs approved for the treatment of hepatitis B. Its safety and lack of significant adverse effects relate to the sparing of mitochondrial DNA and marrow progenitor cells [105]. In nonimmunosuppressed individuals without renal dysfunction, lamivudine has proven efficacy in reducing the level of circulating HBV DNA, improving transaminasemia, and ameliorating hepatic necroinflammatory activity [106, 107].

There is evidence that lamivudine is also effective in dialysis patients and renal allograft recipients, resulting in the suppression of viral replication and aminotransferase normalization in more than 80% of patients (106, 108). After treatment durations lasting 10 to 14 months, lamivudine therapy cleared HBeAg in over 20% of patients, and suppressed HBV DNA to undetectable levels in 50-100%. There is little information on histological changes after treatment in dialysis patients.

However, the selection of drug-resistant variants after prolonged treatment with lamivudine presents a major limitation [109-111]. Such resistance, occurring in around 15% of patients after 12 months, more than 30% after two years, and over half of patients after three years of lamivudine therapy, is almost universally associated with mutations in the highly conserved YMDD (tyrosine, methionine, aspartate, aspartate) nucleotide-binding motif of the major catalytic domain of the HBV RNA dependent DNA polymerase. The emergence of lamivudine resistance can be associated with potentially life-threatening exacerbation of liver disease.

Lamivudine is no longer regarded as the preferred first-line therapy for hepatitis B. In patients without renal disease, entecavir or tenofovir are the recommended first-line oral medications for hepatitis B [112]. It should be noted that tenofovir, similar to adefovir, can lead to renal tubular dysfunction and nephrotoxicity.

Many patients have been treated with lamivudine and have developed drug resistance. For the management of these patients, adefovir add-on therapy has been associated with a high response rate and a lower rate of subsequent resistance compared with switching to adefovir monotherapy [113, 114]. Tenofovir can also be an effective alternative in patients with lamivudine-resistant HBV infection, and has greater antiviral activity compared with adefovir. However, both adefovir and tenofovir are nephrotoxic, and are preferably avoided in dialysis patients with residual renal function, because the latter confers survival benefit.

Switching lamivudine to entecavir monotherapy is also effective in viral suppression, but progressive emergence of entecavir resistance with prolonged treatment could pose a problem [115, 116]. Entecavir is the recommended first-line oral therapy in patients with kidney diseases. The doses of all medications must be adjusted appropriately in patients with end-stage renal disease.

It is recommended that effective treatment be started early after the emergence of lamivudine resistance, both to prevent hepatitic flares and to reduce the risk of subsequent development of multiple drug resistance.

Conclusion

Hepatitis B remains a major health issue in dialysis patients. Despite the introduction of effective infection control measures to minimize patient-to-patient transmission, occasional outbreaks occur in dialysis units, usually due to lapses in practice. In many parts of the world, hepatitis B is endemic and the high background prevalence of the virus is reflected in the dialysis population. An effective vaccine has made a notable contribution to the protection of dialysis patients from the virus, although this is tempered by reduced potency and durability of the anti-HBs response in those with end-stage renal disease. The course of hepatitis B infection is different in patients with dialysis-dependent renal failure. Choosing which patients to treat with antiviral therapy, when, and with which drugs, is a subject of uncertainty at present.

References

[1] Moloughney BW. Transmission and postexposure management of bloodborne virus infections in the health care setting: where are we now? *Cmaj*. [Research Support, U.S. Gov't, P.H.S.Review]. 2001 Aug 21;165(4):445-51.

[2] Lavanchy D. Hepatitis B virus epidemiology, disease burden, treatment, and current and emerging prevention and control measures. *Journal of Viral Hepatitis*. [Review]. 2004 Mar;11(2):97-107.

[3] Dienstag JL. Hepatitis B virus infection. *N. Engl. J. Med.* [Review]. 2008 Oct 2;359(14):1486-500.

[4] Kane M. Global programme for control of hepatitis B infection. *Vaccine*. 1995;13 Suppl 1:S47-9.

[5] Stevens CE, Beasley RP, Tsui J, Lee WC. Vertical transmission of hepatitis B antigen in Taiwan. *N. Engl. J. Med.* [Research Support, U.S. Gov't, Non-P.H.S.]. 1975 Apr 10;292(15):771-4.

[6] Wasley A, Grytdal S, Gallagher K. Surveillance for acute viral hepatitis--United States, 2006. *MMWR Surveill Summ.* 2008 Mar 21;57(2):1-24.

[7] Tassopoulos NC, Papaevangelou GJ, Sjogren MH, Roumeliotou-Karayannis A, Gerin JL, Purcell RH. Natural history of acute hepatitis B surface antigen-positive hepatitis in Greek adults. *Gastroenterology*. [Research Support, Non-U.S. Gov't Research Support, U.S. Gov't, P.H.S.]. 1987 Jun;92(6):1844-50.

[8] Parkin DM, Bray F, Ferlay J, Pisani P. Estimating the world cancer burden: Globocan 2000. *Int. J. Cancer.* 2001 Oct 15;94(2):153-6.

[9] Fabrizi F, Lunghi G, Martin P, Poordad FF. Serological and molecular testing in hepatitis B and the dialysis patient. *Int. J. Artif. Organs.* [Review]. 2002 Feb;25(2):91-9.

[10] Lok AS. Chronic hepatitis B. *N. Engl. J. Med.* [Comment]. 2002 May 30;346(22):1682-3.

[11] London WT, Drew JS, Lustbader ED, Werner BG, Blumberg BS. Host responses to hepatitis B infection in patients in a chronic hemodialysis unit. *Kidney International.* 1977 Jul;12(1):51-8.

[12] Charest AF, McDougall J, Goldstein MB. A randomized comparison of intradermal and intramuscular vaccination against hepatitis B virus in incident chronic hemodialysis patients. *Am. J. Kidney Dis.* [Clinical Trial Randomized Controlled Trial Research Support, Non-U.S. Gov't]. 2000 Nov;36(5):976-82.

[13] Ribot S, Rothstein M, Goldblat M, Grasso M. Duration of hepatitis B surface antigenemia (HBs Ag) in hemodialysis patients. *Arch. Intern.* Med. 1979 Feb;139(2):178-80.

[14] Albertoni F, Battilomo A, Di Nardo V, Franco E, Ippolito G, Marinucci G, et al. Evaluation of a region-wide hepatitis B vaccination program in dialysis patients: experience in an Italian region. The Latium Hepatitis Prevention Group. *Nephron.* 1991;58(2):180-3.

[15] Bruguera M, Rodicio JL, Alcazar JM, Oliver A, Del Rio G, Esteban-Mur R. Effects of different dose levels and vaccination schedules on immune response to a recombinant DNA hepatitis B vaccine in haemodialysis patients. *Vaccine.* [Clinical Trial Randomized Controlled Trial]. 1990 Mar;8 Suppl:S47-9; discussion S60-2.

[16] Steketee RW, Ziarnik ME, Davis JP. Seroresponse to hepatitis B vaccine in patients and staff of renal dialysis centers, Wisconsin. *Am. J. Epidemiol.* 1988 Apr;127(4):772-82.

[17] Kohler H, Arnold W, Renschin G, Dormeyer HH, Meyer zum Buschenfelde KH. Active hepatitis B vaccination of dialysis patients and medical staff. *Kidney International.* 1984 Jan;25(1):124-8.

[18] Rangel MC, Coronado VG, Euler GL, Strikas RA. Vaccine recommendations for patients on chronic dialysis. The Advisory Committee on Immunization Practices and the American Academy of Pediatrics. *Seminars in Dialysis.* [Guideline Practice Guideline]. 2000 Mar-Apr;13(2):101-7.

[19] Waite NM, Thomson LG, Goldstein MB. Successful vaccination with intradermal hepatitis B vaccine in hemodialysis patients previously nonresponsive to intramuscular hepatitis B vaccine. *J. Am. Soc. Nephrol.* 1995 May;5(11):1930-4.

[20] Maisonneuve P, Agodoa L, Gellert R, Stewart JH, Buccianti G, Lowenfels AB, et al. Cancer in patients on dialysis for end-stage renal disease: an international collaborative study. *Lancet.* [Multicenter Study Research Support, Non-U.S. Gov't Research Support, U.S. Gov't, P.H.S.]. 1999 Jul 10;354(9173):93-9.

[21] Marcelli D, Stannard D, Conte F, Held PJ, Locatelli F, Port FK. ESRD patient mortality with adjustment for comorbid conditions in Lombardy (Italy) versus the United States. *Kidney International.* [Comparative Study]. 1996 Sep;50(3):1013-8.

[22] Mathurin P, Mouquet C, Poynard T, Sylla C, Benalia H, Fretz C, et al. Impact of hepatitis B and C virus on kidney transplantation outcome. *Hepatology.* [Clinical Trial]. 1999 Jan;29(1):257-63.

[23] Kliem V, Ringe B, Holhorst K, Frei U. Kidney transplantation in hepatitis B surface antigen carriers. *Clin. Investig.* 1994 Dec;72(12):1000-6.

[24] Parfrey PS, Forbes RD, Hutchinson TA, Kenick S, Farge D, Dauphinee WD, et al. The impact of renal transplantation on the course of hepatitis B liver disease. *Transplantation.* 1985 Jun;39(6):610-5.

[25] Parfrey PS, Farge D, Forbes RD, Dandavino R, Kenick S, Guttmann RD. Chronic hepatitis in end-stage renal disease: comparison of HBsAg-negative and HBsAg-positive patients. *Kidney International.* 1985 Dec;28(6):959-67.

[26] Group RA. Hepatitis and the treatment of chronic renal failure. *Department of Health and social security*, London, UK. 1972.

[27] Control CoD. Hepatitis: control measures for hepatitis B in dialysis centers. HEW publication no. (CDC) 78-8358. US Department of Health *Education and Welfare*, Atlanta, GA. 1977.

[28] Dinits-Pensy M, Forrest GN, Cross AS, Hise MK. The use of vaccines in adult patients with renal disease. *Am. J. Kidney Dis.* [Review]. 2005 Dec;46(6):997-1011.

[29] Desmyter J, Colaert J, De Groote G, Reynders M, Reerink-Brongers EE, Lelie PN, et al. Efficacy of heat-inactivated hepatitis B vaccine in haemodialysis patients and staff. Double-blind placebo-controlled trial. *Lancet.* [Clinical Trial Randomized Controlled Trial Research Support, Non-U.S. Gov't]. 1983 Dec 10;2(8363):1323-8.

[30] Stevens CE, Szmuness W, Goodman AI, Weseley SA, Fotino M. Hepatitis B vaccine: immune responses in haemodialysis patients. *Lancet.* [Clinical Trial Randomized Controlled Trial Research Support, U.S. Gov't, P.H.S.]. 1980 Dec 6;2(8206):1211-3.
[31] Finelli L, Miller JT, Tokars JI, Alter MJ, Arduino MJ. National surveillance of dialysis-associated diseases in the United States, 2002. *Seminars in Dialysis.* [Comparative Study Multicenter Study]. 2005 Jan-Feb;18(1):52-61.
[32] Burdick RA, Bragg-Gresham JL, Woods JD, Hedderwick SA, Kurokawa K, Combe C, et al. Patterns of hepatitis B prevalence and seroconversion in hemodialysis units from three continents: the DOPPS. *Kidney International.* [Multicenter Study Research Support, Non-U.S. Gov't]. 2003 Jun;63(6):2222-9.
[33] Johnson DW, Dent H, Yao Q, Tranaeus A, Huang CC, Han DS, et al. Frequencies of hepatitis B and C infections among haemodialysis and peritoneal dialysis patients in Asia-Pacific countries: analysis of registry data. *Nephrol. Dial. Transplant.* [Comparative Study]. 2009 May;24(5):1598-603.
[34] Carrilho FJ, Moraes CR, Pinho JR, Mello IM, Bertolini DA, Lemos MF, et al. Hepatitis B virus infection in Haemodialysis Centres from Santa Catarina State, Southern Brazil. Predictive risk factors for infection and molecular epidemiology. *BMC Public Health.* [Research Support, Non-U.S. Gov't]. 2004 Apr 27;4:13.
[35] Ferreira RC, Teles SA, Dias MA, Tavares VR, Silva SA, Gomes SA, et al. Hepatitis B virus infection profile in hemodialysis patients in Central Brazil: prevalence, risk factors, and genotypes. *Mem. Inst. Oswaldo Cruz.* [Research Support, Non-U.S. Gov't]. 2006 Sep;101(6):689-92.
[36] Yakaryilmaz F, Gurbuz OA, Guliter S, Mert A, Songur Y, Karakan T, et al. Prevalence of occult hepatitis B and hepatitis C virus infections in Turkish hemodialysis patients. *Renal Failure.* 2006;28(8):729-35.
[37] Wong P-N, Fung T-T, Mak S-K, Lo K-Y, Tong GM, Wong Y, et al. Hepatitis B virus infection in dialysis patients. *Journal of Gastroenterology and Hepatology.* [Review]. 2005;20(11):1641-51.
[38] Bond WW, Favero MS, Petersen NJ, Gravelle CR, Ebert JW, Maynard JE. Survival of hepatitis B virus after drying and storage for one week. *Lancet.* [Letter]. 1981 Mar 7;1(8219):550-1.
[39] Karkar A, Abdelrahman M, Ghacha R, Malik TQ. Prevention of viral transmission in HD units: the value of isolation. *Saudi. J. Kidney Dis. Transpl.* 2006 Jun;17(2):183-8.

[40] Salo RJ, Salo AA, Fahlberg WJ, Ellzey JT. Hepatitis B surface antigen (HBSAg) in peritoneal fluid of HBSAg carriers undergoing peritoneal dialysis. *Journal of Medical Virology*. [In Vitro]. 1980;6(1):29-35.
[41] Oreopoulos DG. Hepatitis and treatment of chronic renal failure by peritoneal dialysis. *Lancet*. 1972 Dec 9;2(7789):1256.
[42] Puttinger H, Vychytil A. Hepatitis B and C in peritoneal dialysis patients. *Seminars in Nephrology*. [Review]. 2002;22(4):351-60.
[43] Hung KY, Shyu RS, Huang CH, Tsai TJ, Chen WY. Viral hepatitis in continuous ambulatory peritoneal dialysis patients in an endemic area for hepatitis B and C infection: the Taiwan experience. *Blood Purification*. [Comparative Study Research Support, Non-U.S. Gov't]. 1997;15(3):195-9.
[44] Tele SA, Martins RM, Lopes CL, dos Santos Carneiro MA, Souza KP, Yoshida CF. Immunogenicity of a recombinant hepatitis B vaccine (Euvax-B) in haemodialysis patients and staff. *Eur. J. Epidemiol.* [Comparative Study Evaluation Studies Research Support, Non-U.S. Gov't]. 2001;17(2):145-9.
[45] Lanini S, Puro V, Lauria FN, Fusco FM, Nisii C, Ippolito G. Patient to patient transmission of hepatitis B virus: a systematic review of reports on outbreaks between 1992 and 2007. *BMC Med.* [Research Support, Non-U.S. Gov't Review]. 2009;7:15.
[46] Outbreaks of hepatitis B virus infection among hemodialysis patients--California, Nebraska, and Texas, 1994. *MMWR Morb. Mortal Wkly. Rep.* 1996 Apr 12;45(14):285-9.
[47] Chu CM, Liaw YF, Pao CC, Huang MJ. The etiology of acute hepatitis superimposed upon previously unrecognized asymptomatic HBsAg carriers. *Hepatology*. [Research Support, Non-U.S. Gov't]. 1989 Mar;9(3):452-6.
[48] Liaw YF, Sheen IS, Chen TJ, Chu CM, Pao CC. Incidence, determinants and significance of delayed clearance of serum HBsAg in chronic hepatitis B virus infection: a prospective study. *Hepatology*. [Research Support, Non-U.S. Gov't]. 1991 Apr;13(4):627-31.
[49] Szmuness W, Stevens CE, Harley EJ, Zang EA, Alter HJ, Taylor PE, et al. Hepatitis B vaccine in medical staff of hemodialysis units: efficacy and subtype cross-protection. *N. Engl. J. Med.* [Clinical Trial Randomized Controlled Trial Research Support, U.S. Gov't, P.H.S.]. 1982 Dec 9;307(24):1481-6.

[50] Tsang TK, Blei AT, O'Reilly DJ, Decker R. Clinical significance of concurrent hepatitis B surface antigen and antibody positivity. *Dig. Dis. Sci.* [Comparative Study Research Support, U.S. Gov't, Non-P.H.S.]. 1986 Jun;31(6):620-4.

[51] Maruyama T, Schodel F, Iino S, Koike K, Yasuda K, Peterson D, et al. Distinguishing between acute and symptomatic chronic hepatitis B virus infection. *Gastroenterology.* [Comparative Study]. 1994 Apr;106(4):1006-15.

[52] Lok AS, Lai CL, Wu PC. Prevalence of isolated antibody to hepatitis B core antigen in an area endemic for hepatitis B virus infection: implications in hepatitis B vaccination programs. *Hepatology.* [Research Support, Non-U.S. Gov't]. 1988 Jul-Aug;8(4):766-70.

[53] Chung HT, Lee JS, Lok AS. Prevention of posttransfusion hepatitis B and C by screening for antibody to hepatitis C virus and antibody to HBcAg. *Hepatology.* [Comparative Study Research Support, Non-U.S. Gov't]. 1993 Nov;18(5):1045-9.

[54] Hoofnagle JH, Seeff LB, Bales ZB, Zimmerman HJ. Type B hepatitis after transfusion with blood containing antibody to hepatitis B core antigen. *N. Engl. J. Med.* [Clinical Trial Randomized Controlled Trial]. 1978 Jun 22;298(25):1379-83.

[55] Dickson RC, Everhart JE, Lake JR, Wei Y, Seaberg EC, Wiesner RH, et al. Transmission of hepatitis B by transplantation of livers from donors positive for antibody to hepatitis B core antigen. The National Institute of Diabetes and Digestive and Kidney Diseases Liver Transplantation Database. *Gastroenterology.* [Research Support, U.S. Gov't, P.H.S.]. 1997 Nov;113(5):1668-74.

[56] McMahon BJ, Parkinson AJ, Helminiak C, Wainwright RB, Bulkow L, Kellerman-Douglas A, et al. Response to hepatitis B vaccine of persons positive for antibody to hepatitis B core antigen. *Gastroenterology.* 1992 Aug;103(2):590-4.

[57] Okada K, Kamiyama I, Inomata M, Imai M, Miyakawa Y. e antigen and anti-e in the serum of asymptomatic carrier mothers as indicators of positive and negative transmission of hepatitis B virus to their infants. *N. Engl. J. Med.* 1976 Apr 1;294(14):746-9.

[58] Beasley RP, Trepo C, Stevens CE, Szmuness W. The e antigen and vertical transmission of hepatitis B surface antigen. *Am. J. Epidemiol.* [Research Support, U.S. Gov't, Non-P.H.S.]. 1977 Feb;105(2):94-8.

[59] Alter HJ, Seeff LB, Kaplan PM, McAuliffe VJ, Wright EC, Gerin JL, et al. Type B hepatitis: the infectivity of blood positive for e antigen and DNA polymerase after accidental needlestick exposure. *N. Engl. J. Med.* 1976 Oct 21;295(17):909-13.

[60] Lok AS, Lai CL. A longitudinal follow-up of asymptomatic hepatitis B surface antigen-positive Chinese children. *Hepatology.* [Research Support, Non-U.S. Gov't]. 1988 Sep-Oct;8(5):1130-3.

[61] Hoofnagle JH, Dusheiko GM, Seeff LB, Jones EA, Waggoner JG, Bales ZB. Seroconversion from hepatitis B e antigen to antibody in chronic type B hepatitis. *Annals of Internal Medicine.* 1981 Jun;94(6):744-8.

[62] Realdi G, Alberti A, Rugge M, Bortolotti F, Rigoli AM, Tremolada F, et al. Seroconversion from hepatitis B e antigen to anti-HBe in chronic hepatitis B virus infection. *Gastroenterology.* 1980 Aug;79(2):195-9.

[63] Bonino F, Rosina F, Rizzetto M, Rizzi R, Chiaberge E, Tardanico R, et al. Chronic hepatitis in HBsAg carriers with serum HBV-DNA and anti-HBe. *Gastroenterology.* [Comparative Study Research Support, Non-U.S. Gov't]. 1986 May;90(5 Pt 1):1268-73.

[64] Lok AS, Hadziyannis SJ, Weller IV, Karvountzis MG, Monjardino J, Karayiannis P, et al. Contribution of low level HBV replication to continuing inflammatory activity in patients with anti-HBe positive chronic hepatitis B virus infection. *Gut.* [Research Support, Non-U.S. Gov't]. 1984 Nov;25(11):1283-7.

[65] Carman WF, Jacyna MR, Hadziyannis S, Karayiannis P, McGarvey MJ, Makris A, et al. Mutation preventing formation of hepatitis B e antigen in patients with chronic hepatitis B infection. *Lancet.* [Comparative Study Research Support, Non-U.S. Gov't]. 1989 Sep 9;2(8663):588-91

[66] Krugman S, Giles JP, Hammond J. Viral hepatitis, type B (MS-2 strain) prevention with specific hepatitis B immune serum globulin. JAMA : *the journal of the American Medical Association.* 1971 Dec 13;218(11):1665-70.

[67] Buynak EB, Roehm RR, Tytell AA, Bertland AU, 2nd, Lampson GP, Hilleman MR. Vaccine against human hepatitis B. JAMA : *the journal of the American Medical Association.* 1976 Jun 28;235(26):2832-4.

[68] Adkins JC, Wagstaff AJ. Recombinant hepatitis B vaccine: a review of its immunogenicity and protective efficacy against hepatitis B. *Bio. Drugs.* 1998 Aug;10(2):137-58.

[69] Zuckerman JN, Sabin C, Craig FM, Williams A, Zuckerman AJ. Immune response to a new hepatitis B vaccine in healthcare workers who had not responded to standard vaccine: randomised double blind dose-response study. *Bmj.* [Clinical Trial Randomized Controlled Trial Research Support, Non-U.S. Gov't]. 1997 Feb 1;314(7077):329-33.

[70] Shepard CW, Simard EP, Finelli L, Fiore AE, Bell BP. Hepatitis B virus infection: epidemiology and vaccination. *Epidemiol. Rev.* [Review]. 2006;28:112-25.

[71] Andre FE. Overview of a 5-year clinical experience with a yeast-derived hepatitis B vaccine. *Vaccine.* [Clinical Trial]. 1990 Mar;8 Suppl:S74-8; discussion S9-80.

[72] McMahon BJ, Helminiak C, Wainwright RB, Bulkow L, Trimble BA, Wainwright K. Frequency of adverse reactions to hepatitis B vaccine in 43,618 persons. *Am. J. Med.* 1992 Mar;92(3):254-6.

[73] Szmuness W, Stevens CE, Harley EJ, Zang EA, Oleszko WR, William DC, et al. Hepatitis B vaccine: demonstration of efficacy in a controlled clinical trial in a high-risk population in the United States. *N. Engl. J. Med.* [Clinical Trial Randomized Controlled Trial Research Support, Non-U.S. Gov't Research Support, U.S. Gov't, P.H.S.]. 1980 Oct 9;303(15):833-41.

[74] Crosnier J, Jungers P, Courouce AM, Laplanche A, Benhamou E, Degos F, et al. Randomised placebo-controlled trial of hepatitis B surface antigen vaccine in french haemodialysis units: II, Haemodialysis patients. *Lancet.* [Clinical Trial Randomized Controlled Trial]. 1981 Apr 11;1(8224):797-800.

[75] Stevens CE, Alter HJ, Taylor PE, Zang EA, Harley EJ, Szmuness W. Hepatitis B vaccine in patients receiving hemodialysis. Immunogenicity and efficacy. *N. Engl. J. Med.* [Clinical Trial Randomized Controlled Trial Research Support, U.S. Gov't, P.H.S.]. 1984 Aug 23;311(8): 496-501.

[76] Grob PJ, Binswanger U, Zaruba K, Joller-Jemelka HI, Schmid M, Hacki W, et al. Immunogenicity of a hepatitis B subunit vaccine in hemodialysis and in renal transplant recipients. *Antiviral Res.* [Comparative Study]. 1983 Mar;3(1):43-52.

[77] Crosnier J, Jungers P, Courouce AM, Laplanche A, Benhamou E, Degos F, et al. Randomised placebo-controlled trial of hepatitis B surface antigen vaccine in French haemodialysis units: I, Medical staff. *Lancet.* [Clinical Trial Randomized Controlled Trial]. 1981 Feb 28;1(8218): 455-9.

[78] Fujiyama S, Yoshida K, Sato T, Shimada H, Deguchi T. Immunogenicity and safety of recombinant yeast-derived hepatitis B vaccine in haemodialysis patients. *Hepato-Gastroenterology.* 1990 Dec;37 Suppl 2:140-4.

[79] Peces R, de la Torre M, Alcazar R, Urra JM. Prospective analysis of the factors influencing the antibody response to hepatitis B vaccine in hemodialysis patients. *American Journal of Kidney Diseases.* 1997;29(2):239-45.

[80] Guan R, Tay HH, Choong HL, Yap I, Woo KT. Hepatitis B vaccination in chronic renal failure patients undergoing haemodialysis: the immunogenicity of an increased dose of a recombinant DNA hepatitis B vaccine. *Ann. Acad. Med. Singapore.* [Comparative Study Research Support, Non-U.S. Gov't]. 1990 Nov;19(6):793-7.

[81] Buti M, Viladomiu L, Jardi R, Olmos A, Rodriguez JA, Bartolome J, et al. Long-term immunogenicity and efficacy of hepatitis B vaccine in hemodialysis patients. *American Journal of Nephrology.* 1992;12(3):144-7.

[82] Agarwal SK, Irshad M, Dash SC. Comparison of two schedules of hepatitis B vaccination in patients with mild, moderate and severe renal failure. *J. Assoc. Physicians India.* [Clinical Trial Comparative Study Controlled Clinical Trial Research Support, Non-U.S. Gov't]. 1999 Feb;47(2):183-5.

[83] DaRoza G, Loewen A, Djurdjev O, Love J, Kempston C, Burnett S, et al. Stage of chronic kidney disease predicts seroconversion after hepatitis B immunization: earlier is better. *Am. J. Kidney Dis.* [Comparative Study]. 2003 Dec;42(6):1184-92.

[84] Evans TG, Schiff M, Graves B, Agosti J, Barritt ML, Garner D, et al. The safety and efficacy of GM-CSF as an adjuvant in hepatitis B vaccination of chronic hemodialysis patients who have failed primary vaccination. *Clinical Nephrology.* [Clinical Trial Randomized Controlled Trial Research Support, Non-U.S. Gov't]. 2000;54(2):138-42.

[85] Jungers P, Devillier P, Salomon H, Cerisier JE, Courouce AM. Randomised placebo-controlled trial of recombinant interleukin-2 in chronic uraemic patients who are non-responders to hepatitis B vaccine. *Lancet.* [Clinical Trial Multicenter Study Randomized Controlled Trial]. 1994 Sep 24;344(8926):856-7.

[86] Miquilena-Colina ME, Lozano-Rodriguez T, Garcia-Pozo L, Saez A, Rizza P, Capone I, et al. Recombinant interferon-alpha2b improves immune response to hepatitis B vaccination in haemodialysis patients: results of a randomised clinical trial. *Vaccine.* [Randomized Controlled Trial Research Support, Non-U.S. Gov't]. 2009;27(41):5654-60.

[87] Quiroga JA, Castillo I, Porres JC, Casado S, Saez F, Gracia Martinez M, et al. Recombinant gamma-interferon as adjuvant to hepatitis B vaccine in hemodialysis patients. *Hepatology.* [Clinical Trial Randomized Controlled Trial]. 1990 Oct;12(4 Pt 1):661-3.

[88] Fabrizi F, Dixit V, Martin P. Meta-analysis: the adjuvant role of thymopentin on immunological response to hepatitis B virus vaccine in end-stage renal disease. *Alimentary Pharmacology and Therapeutics.* [Meta-Analysis Research Support, Non-U.S. Gov't Review]. 2006;23(11):1559-66.

[89] Tong NK, Beran J, Kee SA, Miguel JL, Sanchez C, Bayas JM, et al. Immunogenicity and safety of an adjuvanted hepatitis B vaccine in pre-hemodialysis and hemodialysis patients. *Kidney International.* [Randomized Controlled Trial Research Support, Non-U.S. Gov't]. 2005 Nov;68(5):2298-303.

[90] Kong NCT, Beran J, Kee SA, Miguel JL, Sanchez C, Bayas JM, et al. A new adjuvant improves the immune response to hepatitis B vaccine in hemodialysis patients. *Kidney International.* [Comment Randomized Controlled Trial Research Support, Non-U.S. Gov't]. 2008;73(7):856-62.

[91] Chen W, Gluud C. Vaccines for preventing hepatitis B in health-care workers. *Cochrane Database Syst. Rev.* [Meta-Analysis Review]. 2005(4):CD000100.

[92] Fabrizi F, Dixit V, Magnini M, Elli A, Martin P. Meta-analysis: intradermal vs. intramuscular vaccination against hepatitis B virus in patients with chronic kidney disease. *Alimentary Pharmacology and Therapeutics.* [Meta-Analysis Research Support, Non-U.S. Gov't Review]. 2006 Aug 1;24(3):497-506.

[93] Chau KF, Cheng YL, Tsang DN, Choi KS, Wong KM, Chak WL, et al. Efficacy and side effects of intradermal hepatitis B vaccination in CAPD patients: a comparison with the intramuscular vaccination. *Am. J. Kidney Dis.* [Clinical Trial Comparative Study Randomized Controlled Trial]. 2004 May;43(5):910-7.

[94] Bock M, Barros E, Veronese FJ. Hepatitis B vaccination in haemodialysis patients: a randomized clinical trial. *Nephrology.* [Comparative Study Randomized Controlled Trial Research Support, Non-U.S. Gov't]. 2009 Apr;14(3):267-72.

[95] Barraclough KA, Wiggins KJ, Hawley CM, van Eps CL, Mudge DW, Johnson DW, et al. Intradermal versus intramuscular hepatitis B vaccination in hemodialysis patients: a prospective open-label randomized controlled trial in nonresponders to primary vaccination.[Erratum appears in *Am. J. Kidney Dis.* 2009 Aug;54(2):393 Note: Dosage error in published abstract; MEDLINE/PubMed abstract corrected]. *American Journal of Kidney Diseases.* [Randomized Controlled Trial]. 2009;54(1):95-103.

[96] Fabrizi F, Andrulli S, Bacchini G, Corti M, Locatelli F. Intradermal versus intramuscular hepatitis b re-vaccination in non-responsive chronic dialysis patients: a prospective randomized study with cost-effectiveness evaluation. *Nephrology Dialysis Transplantation.* [Clinical Trial Comparative Study Randomized Controlled Trial Research Support, Non-U.S. Gov't]. 1997;12(6):1204-11.

[97] Weinstein T, Chagnac A, Boaz M, Ori Y, Herman M, Zevin D, et al. Improved immunogenicity of a novel third-generation recombinant hepatitis B vaccine in patients with end-stage renal disease. *Nephron. Clin. Pract.* 2004;97(2):c67-72.

[98] Degott C, Degos F, Jungers P, Naret C, Courouce AM, Potet F, et al. Relationship between liver histopathological changes and HBsAg in 111 patients treated by long-term hemodialysis. *Liver.* 1983 Dec;3(6): 377-84.

[99] Ozdogan M, Ozgur O, Gur G, Boyacioglu S, Ozderin Y, Demirhan B, et al. Histopathological impacts of hepatitis virus infection in hemodialysis patients: should liver biopsy be performed before renal transplantation? *Artificial Organs.* 1997;21(5):355-8.

[100] Fehr T, Ambuhl PM. Chronic hepatitis virus infections in patients on renal replacement therapy. *Nephrology Dialysis Transplantation.* [Editorial Review]. 2004;19(5):1049-53.

[101] Duarte R, Huraib S, Said R, Abdel-Khadir A, Sullivan S, Chaballout A, et al. Interferon-alpha facilitates renal transplantation in hemodialysis patients with chronic viral hepatitis. *American Journal of Kidney Diseases.* [Case Reports]. 1995;25(1):40-5.

[102] Chan TM, Wu PC, Lau JY, Lok AS, Lai CL, Cheng IK. Interferon treatment for hepatitis C virus infection in patients on haemodialysis. *Nephrol. Dial. Transplant.* [Research Support, Non-U.S. Gov't]. 1997 Jul;12(7):1414-9.

[103] Campistol JM, Esforzado N, Martinez J, Rosello L, Veciana L, Modol J, et al. Efficacy and tolerance of interferon-alpha(2b) in the treatment of chronic hepatitis C virus infection in haemodialysis patients. Pre- and post-renal transplantation assessment. *Nephrol. Dial. Transplant.* [Clinical Trial Multicenter Study Randomized Controlled Trial]. 1999 Nov;14(11):2704-9.

[104] Chan TM, Ho SK, Tang CS, Tse KC, Lam MF, Lai KN, et al. Pilot study of pegylated interferon-alpha 2a in dialysis patients with chronic hepatitis C virus infection. *Nephrology.* [Comparative Study Research Support, Non-U.S. Gov't]. 2007 Feb;12(1):11-7.

[105] Regev A, Schiff ER. Drug therapy for hepatitis B. *Adv. Intern. Med.* [Review]. 2001;46:107-35.

[106] Lai CL, Leung N, Teo EK, Tong M, Wong F, Hann HW, et al. A 1-year trial of telbivudine, lamivudine, and the combination in patients with hepatitis B e antigen-positive chronic hepatitis B. *Gastroenterology.* [Clinical Trial Clinical Trial, Phase II Comparative Study Multicenter Study Randomized Controlled Trial Research Support, Non-U.S. Gov't]. 2005 Aug;129(2):528-36.

[107] Dienstag JL, Perrillo RP, Schiff ER, Bartholomew M, Vicary C, Rubin M. A preliminary trial of lamivudine for chronic hepatitis B infection. *N. Engl. J. Med.* [Clinical Trial Randomized Controlled Trial Research Support, Non-U.S. Gov't Research Support, U.S. Gov't, P.H.S.]. 1995 Dec 21;333(25):1657-61.

[108] Chan TM, Fang GX, Tang CS, Cheng IK, Lai KN, Ho SK. Preemptive lamivudine therapy based on HBV DNA level in HBsAg-positive kidney allograft recipients. *Hepatology.* [Clinical Trial Research Support, Non-U.S. Gov't]. 2002 Nov;36(5):1246-52.

[109] Fontaine H, Thiers V, Chretien Y, Zylberberg H, Poupon RE, Brechot C, et al. HBV genotypic resistance to lamivudine in kidney recipients and hemodialyzed patients. *Transplantation.* 2000;69(10):2090-4.

[110] Kletzmayr J, Watschinger B, Muller C, Demetriou D, Puchhammer-Stockl E, Ferenci P, et al. Twelve months of lamivudine treatment for chronic hepatitis B virus infection in renal transplant recipients. *Transplantation.* [Clinical Trial Research Support, Non-U.S. Gov't]. 2000 Nov 15;70(9):1404-7.

[111] Liaw YF, Leung NW, Chang TT, Guan R, Tai DI, Ng KY, et al. Effects of extended lamivudine therapy in Asian patients with chronic hepatitis B. Asia Hepatitis Lamivudine Study Group. *Gastroenterology.* [Clinical Trial Randomized Controlled Trial Research Support, Non-U.S. Gov't]. 2000 Jul;119(1):172-80.
[112] Jafri SM, Lok AS. Antiviral therapy for chronic hepatitis B. *Clin. Liver Dis.* [Research Support, Non-U.S. Gov't Review]. 2010 Aug;14(3): 425-38.
[113] Schiff ER, Lai CL, Hadziyannis S, Neuhaus P, Terrault N, Colombo M, et al. Adefovir dipivoxil therapy for lamivudine-resistant hepatitis B in pre- and post-liver transplantation patients. *Hepatology.* [Multicenter Study Research Support, Non-U.S. Gov't]. 2003 Dec;38(6):1419-27.
[114] Perrillo R, Schiff E, Yoshida E, Statler A, Hirsch K, Wright T, et al. Adefovir dipivoxil for the treatment of lamivudine-resistant hepatitis B mutants. *Hepatology.* [Case Reports]. 2000 Jul;32(1):129-34.
[115] de Man RA, Wolters LM, Nevens F, Chua D, Sherman M, Lai CL, et al. Safety and efficacy of oral entecavir given for 28 days in patients with chronic hepatitis B virus infection. *Hepatology.* [Clinical Trial Randomized Controlled Trial Research Support, Non-U.S. Gov't]. 2001 Sep;34(3):578-82.
[116] Chang TT, Gish RG, Hadziyannis SJ, Cianciara J, Rizzetto M, Schiff ER, et al. A dose-ranging study of the efficacy and tolerability of entecavir in Lamivudine-refractory chronic hepatitis B patients. *Gastroenterology.* [Clinical Trial Multicenter Study Randomized Controlled Trial]. 2005 Oct;129(4):1198-209.

In: Hepatitis B: New Research
Editors: J. T. Cox and D. I. Owen
ISBN 978-1-62081-846-6

Chapter III

Novel Carrier(s) Based Vaccine Design against Hepatitis B: Recent Updates

Rishi Paliwal[1*], Shivani R. Paliwal[2] and Suresh P. Vyas[1]
[1]Drug Delivery Research Laboratory,
Department of Pharmaceutical Sciences,
Dr. H.S. Gour Vishwavidyalaya, Sagar (M.P.), India
[2]SLT Institute of Pharmaceutical Sciences,
Guru Ghasidas Viswavidyalaya, Bilaspur (C.G.), India

Abstract

Strong systemic and long lasting immune response becomes prerequisite when vaccination against hepatitis B is desired. Currently used vaccine for hepatitis B contains one of the viral envelope proteins hepatitis B surface antigens (HBsAg). This strongly evokes humoral immune response and hence protects against the infection. However, cellular immune response which is one of the most important bio-responses that contributes in virus elimination from infected hepatocytes cannot be achieved using conventional vaccine. Although, adjuvant based

* E-mail: rishipaliwal@gmail.com.

vaccination develop strong humoral response but it remains ineffective in generating desired cellular response.

Therefore, to develop a novel and effective vaccine against hepatitis B several strategies including use of carriers based adjuvant system, development of surface functionalized novel antigen carriers and mucosal immunization etc. have been explored. This article describes recent advances in developing novel drug delivery systems based vaccine against hepatitis B.

Keywords: Hepatitis B, Novel Carrier, Adjuvant, Mucosal Immunization

1. Introduction

The Hepatitis B virus (HBV) infection creates severe necroinfalmmatory liver conditions such as liver cirrhosis and hepatocellular carcinomas to the infected person. A large number of HBV carriers are still available for spread of the disease worldwide. For complete eradication of HBV and to remove global fear of this disease, vaccination against this dreadful disease is highly demanded. Conventional hepatitis B vaccine is currently available in the market and is being regularly recommended by clinicians. The conventional approach is based on the use of surface antigen with a dosing schedule of 0, 1 and 6 months respectively. Although the success of this multi dose vaccination is unchallenged, however some other practical problems like parenteral administration, incomplete vaccination due to multi dosing scheduling in large number of cases are some major drawbacks of this vaccine [Aguado 1993, Paliwal *et al.,* 2010].

To solve the latter problem, the requirement of a single dose hepatitis B vaccine was felt and hence to develop such a vaccine several strategies such as use of adjuvant and slow and sustained release of antigen using novel carrier have been explored and evaluated for their desired potential [Bharali *et al.*, 2007, Bharali *et al.*, 2008]. Similarly, parenteral hepatitis B vaccination elicits significantly higher antibody systemic (humoral) response but poor mucosal surface antibody response [Papaevangelou 1998]. Hence, the vaccination remains ineffective being too moderate or insufficient at the mucosal sites in the body which are major ports of HBV entry before its subsequent infection to the liver. Parenteral route of drug delivery is also not preferred route among patients and more specifically among children due to due to associated pain and needle phobia [Nossal 2000]. This is why a needle free single shoot hepatitis B vaccine is needed as an improved hepatitis B vaccine with alternative route of administration [Chadwick *et al.*, 2009, Sanyal and Shi 2009]. Such vaccine should also be clinically effective showing maximum patient compliance with potential of active immunotherapy.

The non-invasive route of administration including mucosal (oral, nasal, rectal etc.) as well as topical route are being consistently explored for development of an effective vaccine against Hepatitis B [Mahor *et al.*, 2007, Davis 2001, Borges *et al.*, 2008, Partidos 2000]. To deliver the antigen at appropriate site of its exploration for effective immunization the designing and optimization of a suitable delivery vehicle is equally important as route of administration. Several carriers such as liposomes, niosomes, nanoparticles etc. are being developed and evaluated for their immunogenic potential using protein as well as DNA based antigens [Lutsiak *et al.*, 1998, Thoelen *et al.*, 2001, Christensen *et al.*, 2011, Chadwick *et al.*, 2009]. The present chapter deals with an aim to review the literature and recent research findings made in order to develop safe and effective vaccine against hepatitis B.

2. Hepatitis B Virus and Vaccination: An Insight

The HBV is a 42 nm sized smallest non-retro viral DNA virus consisted of lipid envelope membrane enclosed icosahedral nucleocapsid protein core having viral DNA and DNA polymerase with reverse transcriptase activity [Tiollais *et al.*, 1985] (Figure 1). HBV is relatively resilient and, in some instances, has been shown to remain infectious on environmental surfaces for more than 7 days at room temperature [Hilleman 1992, Chisari and Ferrari 1995, Hilleman 2003]. Vaccination is a prophylactic therapy which is always considered to be better than treatment of a disease. Severity of an infectious disease like hepatitis B always provoke to scientific community to develop a more effective vaccine [McAuliffe *et al.*, 1980, Fattovich 2003]. At present for vaccination against hepatitis B, a parenteral alum-adsorbed hepatitis B surface antigenic (HBsAg) vaccine is available but has limitation due to serious concerns regarding inability to induce both cell-mediated and mucosal immune response [Gretty 1988].

Historically, the first vaccine against hepatitis B was developed from serum of infected persons. After exposure to HBV, the natural immune system of the body produces anti-HBsAg IgG, which protects such individual from re-infection.

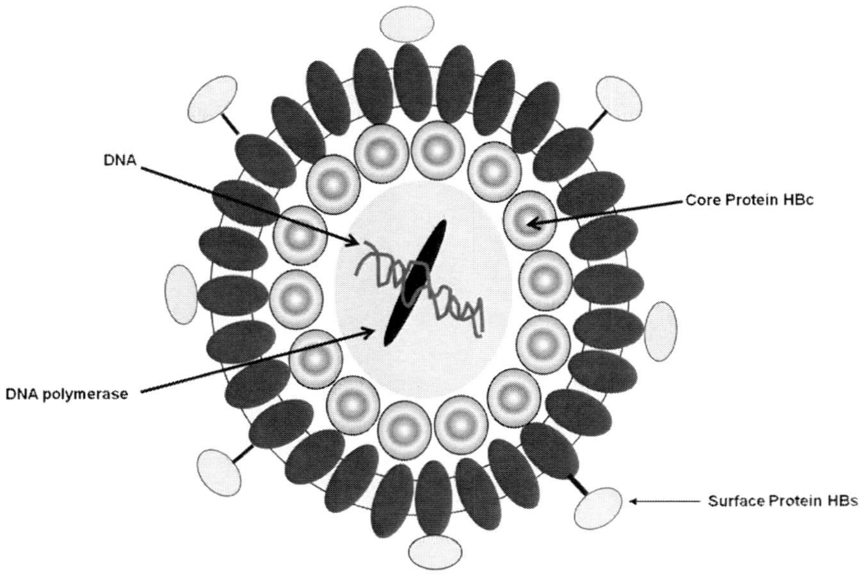

Figure 1. Structure of Hepatitis B Virus (HBV). HBV is 42 nm sized smallest non-retro viral DNA virus consisted of lipid envelope membrane enclosed icosahedral nucleocapsid protein core having viral DNA and DNA polymerase with reverse transcriptase activity. Outer lipid membrane embedded surface protein is known as surface antigen) [Adopted with modifications from Paliwal et al., 2010].

Table 1. List of approaches used for vaccine development against hepatitis B

Formulation of rHBsAg with novel adjuvants	Miscellaneous Approaches	Search of novel antigen in place of rHBsAg
o/w emulsion Microbial derivatives Endogenous immunomodulators Surfactants Lipid based immunomodulators Polymeric micro/nanoparticles	DNA vaccine Combination vaccine Novel adjuvants based formulations Monophosphoryl lipid (MPL) Saponin CpG Oligoneucleotide ISCOMS Liposomes and other novel delivery systems	Synthetic peptide Lipopeptide DNA sequences consisting part of HBV Mutants of HBsAg Hepatitis B core antigen (HBcAg)

The antibodies were collected and purified from blood serum of these infected individuals and subsequently administered to others in order to develop protective immunity. This conventional vaccination approach was not acceptable due to several complications such as shortage of supply and chances of host rejection. Subsequently, it was realized to search other vaccination approaches [Gramzinski *et al.*, 1998]. Outer lipid membrane of HBV embedded surface protein which is known as surface antigen.

It contains several antigenic components, including HBsAg, hepatitis B core antigen (HBcAg), and hepatitis B e antigen (HBeAg) [Chong *et al.*, 2005]. It was observed that in order to develop an efficient hepatitis B vaccine, surface antigen shows promising response in developing protective immune response. Table 1 enlists some of the approaches used for development of hepatitis B vaccine.

3. Mucosal Immunization Against Hepatitis B

A unique advantage of mucosal immunization in generation of immunity at the entry portal surface makes it attractive target for hepatitis B vaccine delivery. The mucosal immune system is guarded by the special lymphoid tissues (mucosally associated lymphoid tissues) for immunity which results in induction of IgA-manifested humoral immunity.

Additionally, cell-mediated immunity can be provoked by the presence of CD4 (+) Th1 and CD8 (+) cells. The immunity generated at the mucosal site is easily transported to the distal mucosal site as well as to systemic pool (Figure 2). Therefore, such understanding of the molecular basis of the mucosal immune system further provides a platform for constructing a mucosal hepatitis B vaccine. The activities of immune system are synergized with co-administration of immunostimulatory molecules. The direct conjugation of antigen with an immunostimulatory molecule or encapsulation it in a ligand anchored carrier can be designed to mimic the receptor-mediated binding of the pathogen. Nanomedicine provided several nanocarriers which have significant contribution in mucosal vaccine development. Mucosal immunization includes oral and nasal immunization as major routes. Topical immunization is also one of the non-invasive approaches hence included for discussion. Table 2 provides key points for comparing parenteral vs mucosal immunization against hepatitis B.

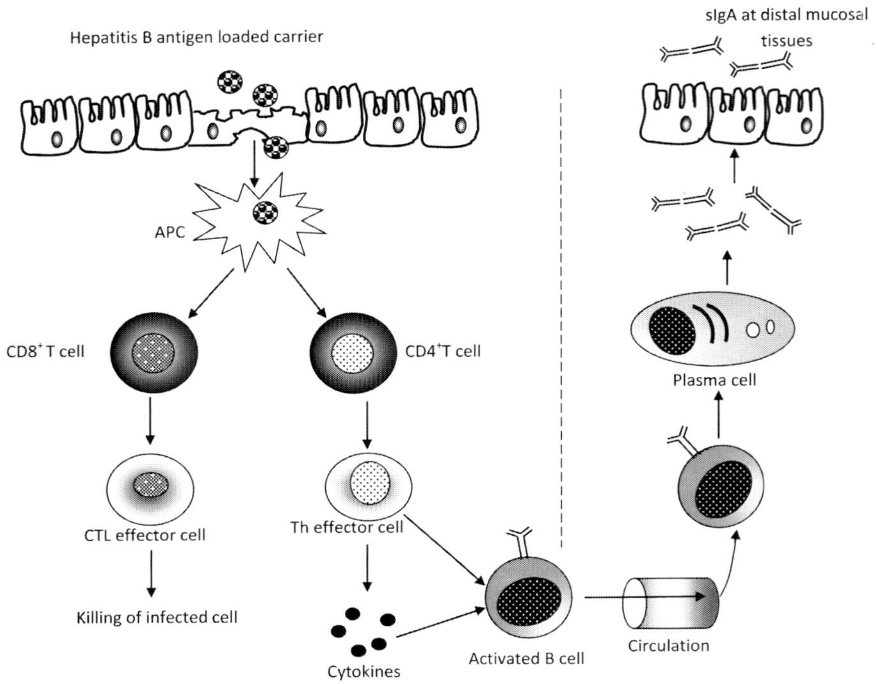

Figure 2. Immune response generation at distant mucosal surfaces followed by mucosal immunization with a hepatitis B antigen loaded novel carrier system [Adopted wih modifications from Paliwal et al., 2010].

3.1. Oral Immunization

Oral antigen delivery may be a prospective solution to the issues associated with conventional vaccination [Simerska *et al.*, 2009]. However, the strategy is detrimental to the antigenic substances and suffers various physical/chemical barriers, and impedes poor transcytosis via mucosal route [Malik *et al.*, 2009]. Transepithelial transport of antigens is the first step in the induction of a mucosal immune response. The delivery of antigens across the epithelial barrier to the underlying lymphoid tissue in GIT is accomplished by M cells [Frey and Neutra 1997]. These specialized cells occur only in the lymphoid follicle-associated epithelium.

To achieve this goal, antigens are coupled to or encapsulated in particulate carriers on to which ligands are being attached to direct it to receptors presents on the M cell surface. Such surface-engineered novel carrier-based approaches are reportedly promising for effective HBsAg oral vaccine delivery [Tiwari and Vyas 2011].

Table 2. Remarkable features of parenteral vs mucoasl immunization against hepatitis B

Objective	Hepatitis B Vaccine Developemnt	
Route of Immunization	Parenteral Immunization (Intramuscular and Subcutaneous)	Mucosal Immunization (Oral, Nasal or Topical)
Advantages	Higher IgG response Immediate access of antigen Antigen stability	Convenient and safe Mimics natural infection Higher mucosal response Ease of administration Targeted immunization to M cells
Limitations	Invasive immunization approach Risk of needle based infection No mucosal protection	Antigen instability High antigen payload
Carriers Exploited	Adjuvant based carriers such as PLGA micro/nanoparticles Liposomes	Liposomes Niosomes Chitosan nanoparticles Lectin anchored liposomes or nanoparticles Trasferosomes Elastic liposomes Bilosomes Alginate coated chitosan nanoparticles

3.2. Nasal Immunization

Nasal vaccination is capable of eliciting strong systemic and local immune responses and is one of the promising routes of needle-free immunization. However, the efficacy of nasally administered antigens is limited due to delivery problems such as easy clearance of free antigens from the nasal cavity, poor absorbtion by nasal epithelial cells and low intrinsic immunogenicity [Slutter *et al.*, 2008]. However, for effective nasal vaccination a critical issue is the antigen-retention period that enables its subsequent interaction with the undelrying lymphatics; further choice of an adjuvant that should be nontoxic in nature but may induce the desired immune response [Debin *et al.*, 2002, Jabbal-Gill 2010]. The encapsulation of the antigen into bio/muco-adhesive nanoparticles is a promising approach towards successful nasal vaccine delivery. These nanoparticles can be engineered by anchoring with targeting ligands, adjuvants or endosomal escape mediators to form the desired vaccine that elicits long-lasting protective immunity [Slutter *et al.*, 2008].

3.3. Topical Immunization

Topical immunisation serves as a convenient and novel approach for vaccination in terms of non-invasiveness and attractive immune cells to generate immunity [Mahor *et al.*, 2007, Paul *et al.*, 1998]. Skin is exploited as a route of immunization because it shows both specific and non-specific immune responses against foreign invaders. The immunocompetent cells within the various skin layers *i.e.* antigen-presenting cells are highly efficient for the initiation of humoral and cellular immune responses. Novel carrier systems including liposomes, vesosomes, niosomes and transferosomes have been widely used for the topical delivery of HBsAg and generate immunity against hepatitis B.

4. Novel Carrier Based Hepatitis B Vaccine

A suitable carrier for vaccine delivery can be defined as representative cargo for loaded antigen to present it safely and effectively at immunologically rich target sites and *vis a vis* act as adjuvant to provoke higher immune response even in smaller doses [Kane 1995]. Numerous nanocarriers including liposomes, niosomes, nanoparticles etc., have been developed for safe and effective delivery of hepatitis B antigens. These carriers are so designed to elicit higher systemic antibody generation and also to generate immune response at different mucosal sites. Table 3 summarizes recent reports on novel carriers used for hepatitis B vaccine development.

4.1. Liposomes

Liposomes are phospholipid bilayered vesicles that can encapsulate protein as well as DNA-based vaccines and offer co-encapsulation of adjuvant along with the antigen.

Table 3. List of reports using novel carrier based immunization against hepatitis B

Route of Immunization	Carrier	Antigen	Remarks	Reference
Parenteral Immunization	MDP derived liposome	rHBsAg	The immunoreactivity of the formulations was found to be effective, leading to a potentially enhanced immune response.	[Jain *et al.*, 2009a]
	LPS-adjuvanted liposome	rHBsAg	LPS-adjuvanted liposomal HBsAg formulations induced stronger cellular immune response with a predominant Interferon-gamma (IFN-gamma) level than those induced by free HBsAg alone, alum-adsorbed HBsAg, and non-adjuvanted liposomal HBsAg.	[Jain *et al.*, 2009b]
	Alginate coated chitosan nanoparticles	rHBsAg, CpG ODN	The enhanced immune response observed with the antigen-loaded nanoparticles and, when co-administered subcutaneously with the CpG ODN, resulted in a mixed Th1/Th2 type immune response.	[Borges *et al.*, 2008]
	Ceramic core based nanodecoy system	rHBsAg	Results indicated that specific anti-HBsAg antibody titers in mice receiving nanodecoy system were more efficient than the conventional adjuvant alum followed by subcutaneous immunization.	[Goyal *et al.*, 2006]
	PLGA microsphere	rHBsAg	A single injection of stabilized HBsAg-PLGA microspheres produced a better immune response than two injections of alum-formulated HBsAg vaccine.	[Jaganathan *et al.*, 2004]

Table 3. (Continued)

Route of Immunization	Carrier	Antigen	Remarks	Reference
	PLA based polymeric lamellar substrate particles	rHBsAg	Immunization with PLSP-rHBsAg resulted in upregulation of specific cellular (lymphoproliferation, IFN-gamma and NO release) as well as IgG response in animals. These responses were higher than those produced by two-dose schedule of alum-adsorbed antigen (alum-rHBsAg).	[Saini *et al.*, 2009]
	Immune stimulating complexes (ISCOMs)	rHBsAg	Immunization with rHBsAg ISCOMs resulted in upregulation of specific cellular (IFN-gamma and IL-2) as well as IgG response (IgG2a isotype biased) humoral response. Immune responses were significantly higher than those produced by of alum-adsorbed antigen (alum-rHBsAg) after (one booster).	[Pandey and Dixit 2009]
	PLGA nanoparticles	Hepatitis B core antigen	The results demonstrated that codelivery of HBcAg and MPLA in PLGA nanoparticles promoted HBcAg-specific Th1 immune responses with IFN-gamma production.	[Chong *et al.*, 2005]

Route of Immunization	Carrier	Antigen	Remarks	Reference
Oral Immunization	PEG-PLA-PEG triblock co-polymeric nanoparticles	rHBsAg	The extent of humoral response obtained in single dose of nanoparticles was comparable to the response produced by alum based vaccine (which received a booster dose) along with better sIgA level at all local and distal mucosal sites.	[Jain *et al.*, 2009]
	Cholera toxin B subunit (CTB) conjugated bilosome	rHBsAg	The system produced anti-HBsAg IgG antibody titre response comparable to that of the intramuscular (IM) injection of 10mug of alum-adsorbed HBsAg.	[Shukla *et al.*, 2010]
	Bilosome	rHBsAg	HBsAg loaded bilosomes produced both systemic as well as mucosal antibody responses upon oral administration. Bilosomes with a five times higher dose upon oral administration produced comparable serum antibody titres to those obtained after intramuscular immunization without the induction of systemic tolerance.	[Shukla *et al.*, 2008]
	Lectin anchored PLGA nanoparticles	rHBsAg	The ligand-coupled nanoparticles demonstrated approximately four folds increase in degree interaction with the BSM as compared to plain nanoparticles. Lectin coupled nanopartilces exhibited enhanced immune response as compared to stabilized non-lectinized nanoparticles.	[Gupta *et al.*, 2006, Gupta *et al.*, 2007]

Table 3. (Continued)

Route of Immunization	Carrier	Antigen	Remarks	Reference
	Manno sylated niosomes	DNA enco ding hepatitis B surface antigen	OPM coated niosomes produced humoral (both systemic and mucosal) and cellular immune response upon oral administration.	[Jain *et al.*, 2005]
	PLGA micro particles	DNA enco ding hepatitis B surface antigen	Oral administration of PLGA-DNA microparticles induced a long-lasting and stable antigen-specific antibody response, both serum total antibody and intestinal IgA. Mice immunized orally exhibited antigen-specific gamma interferon production and cytotoxic T lymphocyte responses in spleen and GALT.	[He *et al.*, 2005]
	Lipodine liposomes	Plasmid DNA pRc/CMV HBS enco ding the S (small) region of hepatitis B surface antigen (HBsAg)	Secreted IgA responses against the encoded HBsAg were substantially higher with liposome-entrapped DNA compared to naked DNA. Expression of the gene, in the draining mesenteric lymph nodes, was much greater in mice dosed with liposomal DNA than in animals dosed with the naked DNA.	[Perrie *et al.*, 2001]
	Chitosan/trimethyl chitosan coated PLGA microparticles	rHBsAg	Coated PLGA particles showed a markedly increased anti-HBsAg titer as compared to plain PLGA microparticles. The results were more pronounced with the TMC-coated PLGA microparticles.	[Pawar *et al.*, 2010]

Route of Immunization	Carrier	Antigen	Remarks	Reference
	PEG-PLA-PEG triblock co-polymeric nanoparticles	rHBsAg	The extent of humoral response obtained in single dose of nanoparticles was comparable to the response produced by alum based vaccine (which received a booster dose) along with better sIgA level at all local and distal mucosal sites.	[Jain *et al.*, 2009]
Nasal Immunization	Chitosan nanoparticles	DNA encoding hepatitis B surface antigen	Chitosan nanoparticles produced humoral and cellular immune responses upon nasal administration.	[Khatri *et al.*, 2008a]
	Chitosan modified liposomes	DNA encoding hepatitis B surface antigen	Glycol chitosan coated liposomes elicited humoral mucosal and cellular immune responses that were significant as compared to naked DNA justifying the potential advantage of mucosal vaccination.	[Khatri *et al.*, 2008b]
	Alginate coated chitosan nanoparticles	rHBsAg, CpG oligodeoxynucleotide	Alginate coated chitosan nanoparticles gave rise to the humoral mucosal immune response. The generation of Th1-biased antigen-specific systemic antibodies and higher interferon-gamma production was observed.	[Borges *et al.*, 2008]
	Chitosan modified PLGA microspheres	rHBsAg	Modified PLGA microspheres (cationic microspheres) produced humoral (both systemic and mucosal) and cellular immune responses upon nasal administration.	[Jaganathan and Vyas 2006]

Table 3. (Continued)

Route of Immunization	Carrier	Antigen	Remarks	Reference
	Cationic emulsion	pCMV-S coding for Hepatitis B virus surface antigen (HBsAg)	Cationic emulsion dramatically enhanced HBsAg expression. Immune response was associated with increases in the levels of HBs-specific Abs in serum and mucosal fluids, of CTL in the spleen and cervical and iliac lymph nodes, and of delayed-type hypersensitivity (DTH) against HBsAg.	[Kim *et al.*, 2006]
	Cationic nano particles (SMBV)	rHBsAg	The detection of a CTL response and an increase in both IgG1 and IgG2a antibodies in serum suggested that SMBV amplifies both Th1 and Th2 responses without modifying the Th1/Th2 profile of the immune response induced by the natural protein.	[Debin *et al.*, 2002]
	Immune stimulating complexes (ISCOMs)	rHBsAg	Serum anti-HBsAg IgG titer after three high nasal doses of ISCOMs was comparable with titer recorded after alum-HBsAg administered subcutaneously. Similarly, modest but higher cellular response (cytokines level in spleen homogenates) and significantly higher secretory sIgA response in mucosal secretions was observed in case of HBsAg ISCOM vaccines.	[Pandey and Dixit 2009]

Route of Immunization	Carrier	Antigen	Remarks	Reference
Topical Immunization	Cationic transferosome	DNA encoding hepatitis B surface antigen	Topical application of DNA loaded cationic transfersomes elicited a comparable serum antibody titer and endogenous cytokines levels as produced after intramuscular recombinant HBsAg administration.	[Mahor *et al.*, 2007]
	Cationic deformable liposomes	DNA encoding hepatitis B surface antigen	It was observed that deformable liposome elicited a comparable serum antibody titre and endogenous cytokines levels compared to other vaccinations.	[Wang *et al.*, 2007]
	Niosome	DNA encoding hepatitis B surface antigen	Topical niosomes elicited a comparable serum antibody titer and endogenous cytokines levels as compared to intramuscular recombinant HBsAg and topical liposomes.	[Vyas *et al.*, 2005]

The use of liposomes as vaccine delivery systems is evolving rapidly owing to the combined increase in technological advances and understanding of the immune system. In recent years, liposome vaccine technology has gained much attention and now several vaccines containing liposome-based adjuvants have been clinically proven to be very effective at pre-clinical and clinical level. Liposomes conatining immunostimulators and antigens have been developed to target diseases that require stimulation of both humoral and cell-mediated immune responses [Henriksen-Lacey *et al.* 2011].

Additionally, surface modified ligand-conjugated liposomes, which are capable for interaction of antigen with the cells of the mucosal immune system, serve as suitable candidates for the mucosal delivery of vaccines. Before exploring Liposome-based vaccines for hepatitis B, it becomes important to understand precisely the mechanism of liposomes interaction with the immune system and stimulation of immunity.

The physicochemical properties of liposomal vaccines - method of antigen attachment, lipid composition, bilayer fluidity, particle charge, and other properties - exert dramatic effects on the resulting immune response [Watson *et al.* 2012]. The latter one has been extensively investigated. Cationic liposomes have also been investigated as vaccine delivery systems and adjuvants. However, cationic liposomes have limited immunostimulatory effect alone hence the combination of liposomes with immunostimulating ligands has arisen as a strategy in the development of novel adjuvant systems. Recently, two novel adjuvant systems based on cationic liposomes incorporating Toll-like receptor or non-Toll-like receptor immunostimulating ligands have been tested. Similarly, a number of new cationic liposome-forming surfactants with notable immunostimulatory properties have been discovered. Interested readers are suggested to read an interesting article written by Christensen *et al.*, 2011 related to the progress on the application of cationic liposomes as vaccine delivery systems/adjuvants [Christensen *et al.* 2011]. Some of the recent reports based on liposome based hepatitis b vaccines are discussed.

Jain *et al.*, 2008 evaluated hepatitis B surface antigen loaded liposomes adjuvanted with rough lipopolysaccharide (Re-LPS) and lpxL1 LPS. They proposed that serum IgG titer obtained after i.m administration of Re-LPS- and lpxL1 LPS-adjuvanted liposomal HBsAg formulation was equivalent to alum-adsorbed HBsAg formulation but was more responsive, sustained, and significantly higher than the corresponding liposomal HBsAg and plain HBsAg formulations. Incorporation of lpxL1 LPS into the liposomal HBsAg increased the stimulation index (SI) 6-10 times as compared with plain

HBsAg. Re-LPS- and lpxL1 LPS-adjuvanted liposomal HBsAg formulations induced stronger cellular immune response with a predominant Interferon-gamma (IFN-gamma) level than those induced by free HBsAg alone, alum-adsorbed HBsAg, and non-adjuvanted liposomal HBsAg. Probably, the possible mechanism for the enhancement of cellular immunity in addition to humoral immunity by LPS-adjuvanted liposomal HBsAg formulation is due to marked enhancement of immunological presentation and recruitment of antigen via macrophage and antigen-presenting cells (APCs) [Jain *et al.*, 2008].

The characterization of immunological cascades of the innate immune system activated by invariant molecular structures termed as pathogen-associated molecular patterns recognized by pattern recognition receptors of macrophages and dendritic cells, have allowed the elucidation of the mechanisms underlying the immunomodulatory properties of adjuvants. In their subsequent study, the same group exploited adjuvant-active lipophilic analogues of N-acetyl muramyl dipeptide (MDP) for development of effective hepatitis b vaccine.

The MDP was incorporated in liposomal hepatitis B surface antigen (HBsAg) formulations. The serum IgG and anti-HBs titer obtained after intramuscular administration of liposomal muramyl tripeptide-phosphatidyl-ethanolamine (MTP-PE) and liposomal N-acetylmuramyl-l-alanyl-diso-glutamine-glycerol dipalmitate (MDP-GDP) antigenic formulations were significantly higher. The incorporation of MTP-PE on the liposomal HBsAg increased the stimulation index (SI) four to five times as compared to plain HBsAg solution, and it also induced significantly higher Th1 cellular immune response with a predominant IFN-gamma level. This novel effective and potentially safe approach in which liposomes act as delivery vehicles for hepatitis B viral antigen to antigen-presenting cells was proposed which could ornamented with a biological response modifier and activated these target cells to enhance the antigen presentation to T lymphocytes. [Jain *et al.*, 2009].

Recently, our group investigated for prospective of recombinantly expressed influenza surface protein haemagglutinin (HA) complexed liposomes for intranasal delivery of HBsAg. Liposomes encapsulating HBsAg were complexed with HA. A significant and perdurable immune response was obtained following in vivo administration of the developed formulations that was comparable with alum adsorbed HBsAg administered intramuscularly. The HA complexed liposomal formulations elicited sIgA in mucosal secretions and also demonstrated cellular immune response both of which are not induced in the case of alum adsorbed HBsAg vaccine. Further, the HA complexed liposomes produced higher immune response as compared to plain liposomes that might be due to higher uptake of former as evidenced in microscopy study of nasal tissues. The higher cellular response generated by HA complexed liposomes may be possibly due to characteristic pH dependent fusion property of HA [Tiwari *et al.* 2011].

The hepatitis B surface antigen (HBsAg) encapsulated liposomes coupled with Ulex europaeus agglutinin 1 (UEA-1) were prepared with an intesion to increase transmucosal uptake by M-cells of the Peyer's patches. It was reportted that lectinized liposomes exibited increased activity with BSM as compared to non-lectinized liposomes and α-l-fucose specificity. The lectinized liposomes targteted M-cells provoked higher serum anti-HBsAg IgG titre obtained after 3 consecutive days oral immunizations with HBsAg encapsulated lectinized liposomes and boosting after third week was comparable with the titre recorded after single intramuscular prime and third week boosting with alum-HBsAg. At the same time, higher sIgA level in mucosal secretions and cytokines level in the spleen homogenates was elicited [Gupta and Vyas 2011].

4.2. PLGA Micro/Nano-particles

Poly (lactide-co-glycolide) acid (PLGA) is one the most widely explored biomaterial in drug delivery and vaccine science [Feng *et al.*, 2005, Feng *et al.*, 2006]. However, no commercial PLGA based vaccine reached to market yet. PLGA microparticles as commercial vaccines are unsucessful due to the instability of encapsulated antigen [Vyas and Gupta 2007]. Over the years, several advancements have been made towards maintaining antigen integrity within PLGA microparticle preparation [Jain *et al.*, 2011]. Some of the recent reports related to PLGA based hepatitis B vaccine design are summarized below.

Shi *et al.* 2002 developed a single-shot Hepatitis B vaccine formulation using poly(d,l)-lactide-co-glycolide acid (PLGA) microspheres as a delivery system. PLGA microsphere successfully encapsulated Hepatitis B surface antigen (HBsAg), a lipoprotein particle with favorable results such as good recoveries of protein mass, protein particle conformational integrity, and in vitro antigenicity. Some partial delipidation of the HBsAg, however, was observed. The immunogenicity of the microsphere formulations of HBsAg was compared with conventional aluminum adjuvant formulated HBsAg vaccine in C3H mice. Comparisons were made between aluminum formulations (one and two injections), PLGA microsphere formulations (single injection), and a mixture of aluminum and PLGA microsphere formulations (single injection). The nine-month serum antibody titers indicated that a single injection of a mixture of aluminum and PLGA-formulated HBsAg results in equal or better immune responses than two injections of aluminum-formulated HBsAg vaccine. It was proposed that HBsAg can be successfully encapsulated and recovered from the PLGA microspheres and a mixture of aluminum-adjuvanted and PLGA-formulated HBsAg can auto-boost an immune response in manner comparable to multiple injections of an aluminum-formulated vaccine [Shi *et al.* 2002].

Jaganathan *et al.* 2004 developed a stable single-dose vaccine based on recombinant hepatitis B surface antigen (HBsAg) in poly(D,L-lactic-co-glycolic acid) (PLGA) microspheres, in which HBsAg was stabilized by a protein stabilizer (trehalose) and an antacid (Mg(OH)2).

To neutralize the acids liberated by the biodegradable lactic/glycolic acid based polymer, the co-incorporation of an antacid, Mg(OH)2, into the polymer which neutralized the acidity during degradation of the polymer and also prevented HBsAg structural losses and aggregation was proposed. A high antigen integrity after encapsulation was confirmed by various techniques like sodium dodecyl sulfate polyacrylamide gel electrophoresis followed by silver staining, isoelectric focusing and Western blotting techniques, which confirmed that antigen remained intact after encapsulation. The release of antigen was found to be improved by the protein stabilizer (trehalose). A single injection of stabilized HBsAg-PLGA microspheres produced a better immune response than two injections of alum-formulated HBsAg vaccine. They highlighted that recombinant HBsAg can be stabilized by use of a protein stabilizer and antacid during entrapment, and this stabilized preparation can be useful for antigen delivery [Jaganathan *et al.* 2004].

Recently, Saini *et al.*, 2011, reported to develop a "single-shot" HBsAg adsorbed microspheres of poly (DL)-lactide-co-glycolide (PLGA) (L/G 50:50 and 75:25) and their capability to stimulate the cell mediated immune response against hepatitis B surface antigen.

The immune-stimulating activities following subcutaneous injection of HBsAg adsorbed PLGA microspheres (single-dose on day 0) suggested superiority of developed formulations over alum adsorbed vaccines (two-doses on 0 and 28 days) in Balb/c mice. They suggested the high capability of cationic polymeric microspheres based vaccine in stimulating cell mediated immune response along with humoral response against hepatitis B. Surface-modified DL-lactide/glycolide copolymer (PLGA) microspheres with chitosan

(CS) developed for nasal immunization using recombinant Hepatitis B (HBsAg) surface protein for the induction of humoral, cellular and mucosal immunity are reported.

The modified PLGA microspheres were having the lowest nasal clearance rate when compared with unmodified PLGA microspheres and lactose powder. The serum anti-HBsAg titre obtained after nasal administration of modified PLGA microspheres was comparable with titre recorded after alum-HBsAg was administered subcutaneously. Moreover, alum-HBsAg vaccine did not elicit sIgA in mucosal secretions as it was induced and measured in the case of nasal administration of modified PLGA microspheres.

Modified PLGA microspheres (cationic microspheres) thus produced humoral (both systemic and mucosal) and cellular immune responses upon nasal administration. Modified PLGA microspheres and their use as a carrier adjuvant for nasal subunit vaccines were justified by such results [Jaganathan and Vyas 2006].

4.3 Chitosan Nanoparticles

Prego *et al.,* 2010, developed polysaccharidic-based nanoparticles as delivery structures for virus-like particle antigens, using recombinant hepatitis B surface antigen (rHBsAg) as a model. These CS-based nanoparticles allowed the efficient association of the antigen (>60%) while maintaining the antigenic epitope intact.

The immunization studies showed the induction of important sero-protection rates after intramuscular administration of the nanoparticles, indicating their adjuvant capacity. In fact, CS-based nanoparticles were able to induce anti-HBsAg IgG levels up to 5500 mIU/ml, values 9-fold the conventional alum-adsorbed vaccine [Prego *et al.,* 2010].

Alginate coated chitosan nanoparticles loaded with the recombinant hepatitis B surface antigen (HBsAg) with the aim of protecting the antigen, adsorbed on the surface of those chitosan nanoparticles, from enzymatic degradation at mucosal surfaces admnistred via intranasal route were reported. The association of HBsAg with the alginate coated chitosan nanoparticles, administered intranasally to the mice, gave rise to the humoral mucosal immune response. Wheras, humoral systemic immune response was not induced by the HBsAg loaded nanoparticles alone [Borges *et al.*, 2008].

4.4. Bilosomes

The use of bile salt stabilized vesicles (bilosomes) for oral HBsAg antigen delivery providing both the protection to the antigen as well as enable transmucosal uptake and subsequent immunization are also reported by our group. The immunization dose using bilosomes that could produce serum antibody titres against hepatitis B via the oral route compared to those following intramuscular immunization were also assesed [Shukla *et al.*, 2008].

The conjugation of bilosomal system with cholera toxin B subunit (CTB) to increase transmucosal uptake via M-cell specific delivery approach was also studied. The results showed that CTB1 produced anti-HBsAg IgG antibody titre response comparable to that of the intramuscular (i.m.) injection of 10 microg of alum-adsorbed HBsAg. Moreover, all the bilosomal preparations elicited measurable sIgA vis-à-vis negligible response with i.m. administered HBsAg. These results confirmed that HBsAg-loaded CTB-conjugated bilosomes provide a promising potential for targeted oral immunization against hepatitis B [Shukla *et al.*, 2010].

4.5. Niosomes

Niosomes are non-ionic surfactant vesicles obtained on hydration of synthetic nonionic surfactants, with or without incorporation of cholesterol or other lipids. They are vesicular systems similar to liposomes that can be used as carriers of amphiphilic and lipophilic drugs. Though, liposomes have been widely employed for DNA delivery through topical route; however, they suffer from certain drawbacks like higher cost and instability. Non-ionic surfactant based vesicles (niosomes) for topical delivery of DNA encoding hepatitis B surface antigen (HBsAg) has been reported. It was claimed that topical niosomes elicited a comparable serum antibody titer and endogenous cytokines levels as compared to intramuscular recombinant HBsAg and topical liposomes.

Niosomes coated with a modified polysaccharide o-palmitoyl mannan (OPM) were also reported in order to protect them from bile salt caused dissolution and enzymatic degradation in the gastrointestinal tract and to enhance their affinity towards the antigen presenting cells of Peyer's patches [Jain *et al.*, 2005]. OPM coated niosomes were found to better stable in simulated GIT conditions. The serum anti-HBsAg titer obtained after oral administration of OPM coated niosomal formulations to mice was although less as compared to that elicited by naked DNA and pure HBsAg administered intramuscularly, but the mice were seroprotective within 2 weeks and antibody level far above the clinically protective limit for humans was achieved. Similarly, cellular response (cytokines level) was absent in pure HBsAg treated animals. OPM coated niosomes produced humoral (both systemic and mucosal) and cellular immune response upon oral administration.

4.6. Transferosomes

Transferosome are also known as ultrafelexible liposomes. These carriers are composed of lipid which self-assembles into lipid bilayer as in case of conventional liposomes. By addition bilayer softening component, lipid bilayer flexibility and permeability is altered. This is how these vesicles can adapt its shape easily according to the need by adjusting local conentration of each layer component to the local stress experienced by the bilayer.

A novel modified version of transfersomes, i.e., cationic transfersomes for topical DNA vaccine delivery was reported by our group. Plasmid DNA encoding hepatitis B surface antigen (HBsAg) was loaded in the cationic transfersomes using charge neutralization method. Results of this studies revealed that DNA loaded cationic transfersomes elicited significantly higher anti-HBsAg antibody titer and cytokines level as compared to naked DNA. It was also observed that topical application of DNA loaded cationic transfersomes elicited a comparable serum antibody titer and endogenous cytokines levels as produced after intramuscular recombinant HBsAg administration [Mahor *et al.*, 2007]. Mishra *et al.*, 2006 reported elastic liposomes for transcutaneous delivery Hepatitis B surface antigen (HBsAg) to enhance immunity against the antigen. Transcutaneous immunization via elastic liposomes could induce robust systemic and mucosal antibody response against HBsAg. A prominent skin permeation and biodistribution of elastic liposomes, demonstrating efficient delivery of antigens to the immunocompetent Langerhans cells (LC) and lymphatics was also claimed (Mishra *et al.* 2006, Mishra *et al.*, 2007, Mishra *et al.*, 2008). In another similar report, hepatitis B surface antigen (HBsAg) plasmid DNA-cationic complex deformable liposome was used to enhance immunity. These deformable liposomes elicited a comparable serum antibody titre and endogenous cytokines levels compared to other vaccination and demonstrated potential of deformable liposome as DNA vaccine carriers for effective transcutaneous immunization [Wang *et al.*, 2007].

Conclusion

The molecular understanding of immunological bio-events is rapidly growing with advancement of newer technologies. Therefore, selective localization/delivery of antigen by using novel carrier(s) systems is expected to develop new generation hepatitis B vaccine. Major challenges in the development of such new generation against chronic hepatitis B virus infection are induction of potent cellular immune responses and the efficient targeting of the antigen to specific immune cells. The encapsulation of HBsAg antigen into an engineered nanocarrier arisen as the future options. However, stimulation of immune response with single dose administration using non-invasive routes of delivery and using appropriately designed carrier system will serve as an ideal approach for cost-effective vaccine against hepatitis B.

References

Aguado, M.T. (1993). Future approaches to vaccine development: single-dose vaccines using controlled release delivery systems. *Vaccine*, 11, 596–597.

Bharali, D.J.; Mousa, S.A.; Thanavala, Y. (2007). Micro- and nanoparticle-based vaccines for hepatitis B. *Adv. Exp. Med. Biol.*, 601, 415-421.

Bharali; D.J., Pradhan, V.; Elkin, G. *et al.* (2008). Novel nanoparticles for the delivery of recombinant hepatitis B vaccine. *Nanomedicine*, 4, 311-317.

Borges, O.; Cordeiro-da-Silva, A.; Tavares, J.; Santarém, N.; de Sousa, A.; Borchard, G.; Junginger, H.E. (2008). Immune response by nasal delivery of hepatitis B surface antigen and codelivery of a CpG ODN in alginate coated chitosan nanoparticles. *Eur. J. Pharm. Biopharm.*, 69, 405-416.

Chadwick, S.; Kriegel, C.; Amiji, M. (2009). Nanotechnology solutions for mucosal immunization. *Adv. Drug. Deliv. Rev*. 62, 394-407.

Chisari, F.V.; Ferrari, C. (1995). Hepatitis B virus immunopathogenesis. *Annu. Rev. Immunol.,* 13, 29–60.

Chong, C.S.; Cao, M.; Wong, W.W. *et al.* (2005) Enhancement of T helper type 1 immune responses against hepatitis B virus core antigen by PLGA nanoparticle vaccine delivery. *J. Control Release,* 102, 85-99.

Christensen, D.; Korsholm, K.S.; Andersen, P.; Agger, E.M. (2011). Cationic liposomes as vaccine adjuvants. *Expert Rev. Vaccines,* 2011, 10, 513-521.

Davis, S.S. (2001). Nasal Vaccines. *Adv. Drug Deliv. Rev.,* 51, 21-42.

Debin, A.; Kravtzoff, R.; Santiago, J.V.; *et al.* (2002). Intranasal immunization with recombinant antigens associated with new cationic particles induces strong mucosal as well as systemic antibody and CTL responses. *Vaccine*, 20, 2752-2763.

Fattovich, G. (2003). Natural history of hepatitis B. *J. Hepatol.,* 39, S50-58.

Feng, L.; Qi, X.R., Zhou, X.J.; *et al.* (2006). Pharmaceutical and immunological evaluation of a single-dose hepatitis B vaccine using PLGA microspheres. *J. Control Release,* 112, 35-42.

Feng, L.; Zhou, X.J.; Qi, X.R. (2005). Preparation, release and immunogenicity evaluation of HBsAg-PLGA microspheres. *Beijing Da Xue Xue Bao*, 37, 527-531.

Feng, L.; Zhou, X.J.; Wang, S.C.; Jiang, Y.; Qi, X.R. (2006). Immunogenicity of single-dose HBsAg-PLGA controlled release microspheres in mice. *Yao Xue Xue Bao*, 41, 132-137.

Frey, A.; Neutra, M.R. (1997). Targeting of mucosal vaccines to Peyer's patch M cells. *Behring. Inst. Mitt.*, 98, 376-389.

Goyal, A.K.; Rawat, A.; Mahor, S.; Gupta, P.N.; Khatri, K.; Vyas, S.P. (2006). Nanodecoy system: a novel approach to design hepatitis B vaccine for immunopotentiation. *Int. J. Pharm.,* 309, 227-233.

Gramzinski, R.A.; Millan, C.L.; Obaldia, N.; Hoffman, S.L.; Davis, H.L. (1998). Immune response to a hepatitis B DNA vaccine in Aotus monkeys: a comparison of vaccine formulation, route, and method of administration. *Mol. Med.,* 4, 109-118.

Gretty, R.J. Recombinant hepatitis B vaccines. In: Zuckerman, A.J.; Alan, R. (Editors). *Viral hepatitis and liver disease.* New York; 1988; 1017-1024.

Gupta, P.N.; Khatri, K.; Goyal, A.K.; Mishra, N.; Vyas, S.P. (2007). M-cell targeted biodegradable PLGA nanoparticles for oral immunization against hepatitis B. *J. Drug Target,* 15, 701-713.

Gupta, P.N.; Mahor, S.; Rawat, A.; Khatri, K.; Goyal, A.; Vyas, S.P. (2006). Lectin anchored stabilized biodegradable nanoparticles for oral immunization 1. Development and in vitro evaluation. *Int. J. Pharm.,* 318, 163-173.

He, X.W.; Wang, F.; Jiang, L.; *et al.* (2005). Induction of mucosal and systemic immune response by single-dose oral immunization with biodegradable microparticles containing DNA encoding HBsAg. *J. Gen. Virol.,* 86, 601-610.

Henriksen-Lacey, M.; Korsholm, K.S.; Andersen, P.; Perrie, Y.; Christensen, D. (2011). Liposomal vaccine delivery systems. *Expert Opin. Drug Deliv.,* 2011, 8, 505-519.

Hilleman, M.R. (2003). Critical overview and outlook: pathogenesis, prevention and treatment of hepatitis and hepatocarcinoma caused by hepatitis B virus. *Vaccine,* 21, 4626-4649.

Hilleman, M.R. (1992). Plasma-derived hepatitis B vaccine-a breakthrough in preventive medicine. In: Ellis, RW, editor. *Hepatitis B Vaccines in Clinical Practice.* New York: 1992; 17-39.

Jabbal-Gill, I. (2010). Nasal vaccine innovation. *J. Drug Target*, 2010, 18, 771-86.

Jaganathan, K.S.; Singh, P.; Prabakaran, D.; Mishra, V.; Vyas, S.P. (2004). Development of a single-dose stabilized poly (D, L-lactic-co-glycolic acid) microspheres-based vaccine against hepatitis B. *J. Pharm. Pharmacol.,* 56, 1243-1250.

Jaganathan, K.S.; Vyas, S.P. (2006). Strong systemic and mucosal immune responses to surface-modified PLGA microspheres containing recombinant hepatitis B antigen administered intranasally. *Vaccine*, 24, 4201-4211.

Jain, A.K.; Goyal, A.K.; Gupta, P.N.; Khatri, K.; Mishra, N.; Mehta, A.; Mangal, S.; Vyas, S.P. (2009). Synthesis, characterization and evaluation of novel triblock copolymer based nanoparticles for vaccine delivery against hepatitis B. J. Control Release, 136, 161-169.

Jain, A.K.; Goyal, A.K.; Mishra, N.; Vaidya, B.; Mangal, S.; Vyas, S.P. (2010). PEG-PLA-PEG block copolymeric nanoparticles for oral immunization against hepatitis B. *Int. J. Pharm.,* 387, 253-262.

Jain, S.; Singh, P.; Mishra, V.; Vyas, S.P. (2005). Mannosylated niosomes as adjuvant-carrier system for oral genetic immunization against hepatitis B. *Immunol. Lett.,* 101, 41-49.

Jain, S.; O'Hagan, D.T.; Singh, M. (2011). The long-term potential of biodegradable poly (lactide-co-glycolide) microparticles as the next-generation vaccine adjuvant. *Expert Rev. Vaccines*. 10, 1731-1742.

Jain, V.; Sahu, R.; Misra-Bhattacharya, S.; Vyas, S.P.; Kohli, D. (2008). Enhancement of T-helper type I immune responses against hepatitis B surface antigen by LPS derivatives adjuvanted liposomes delivery system. *J. Drug Target,* 6, 706-715.

Jain, V.; Vyas, S.P.; Kohli, D.V. (2009). Well-defined and potent liposomal hepatitis B vaccines adjuvanted with lipophilic MDP derivatives. *Nanomedicine*. 5, 334-344.

Kane, M. (1995). Reduced doses of hepatitis B vaccines: is it a good idea? *Bull World Health Organ*, 73, 529-530.

Khatri, K.; Goyal, A.K.; Gupta, P.N.; Mishra, N.; Mehta, A.; Vyas, S.P. (2008). Surface modified liposomes for nasal delivery of DNA vaccine. *Vaccine*, 26, 2225-2233.

Khatri, K.; Goyal, A.K.; Gupta, P.N.; Mishra, N.; Vyas, S.P. (2008). Plasmid DNA loaded chitosan nanoparticles for nasal mucosal immunization against hepatitis B. *Int. J. Pharm.,* 354, 235-241.

Kim, T.W.; Chung, H.; Kwon, I.C.; *et al.* (2006). Induction of immunity against hepatitis B virus surface antigen by intranasal DNA vaccination using a cationic emulsion as a mucosal gene carrier. *Mol. Cells,* 22, 175-181.

Lutsiak, C.M.; Sosnowski, D.L.; Wishart, D.S.; Kwon, G.S.; Samuel, J. (1998). Use of a liposome antigen delivery system to alter immune responses in vivo. *J. Pharm. Sci.,* 87, 1428-1432.

Mahor, S.; Gupta, P.N.; Rawat, A.; Vyas, S.P. (2007). A needle-free approach for topical immunization: antigen delivery via vesicular carrier system(s). *Curr. Med. Chem.,* 14, 2898-2910.

Mahor, S.; Rawat, A.; Dubey, P.K.; *et al.* (2007). Cationic transfersomes based topical genetic vaccine against hepatitis B. *Int. J. Pharm.,* 340, 13-19.

Malik, B.; Goyal, A.K.; Mangal, S.; Zakir, F.; Vyas, S.P. (2010). Implication of Gut Immunology in the Design of Oral Vaccines. *Curr. Mol. Med.,* 10, 47-70.

McAuliffe, V.J.; Purcell, R.H.; Gerin, J.L. (1980). Type B hepatitis: a review of current prospects for a safe and effective vaccine. *Rev. Infect. Dis.,* 2, 470-492.

Mishra, D.; Dubey, V.; Asthana, A.; Saraf, D.K.; Jain, N.K. (2006). Elastic liposomes mediated transcutaneous immunization against Hepatitis B. *Vaccine,* 24, 4847-4855.

Mishra, D.; Mishra, P.K.; Dubey, V.; Dabadghao, S.; Jain, N.K. (2007). Evaluation of uptake and generation of immune response by murine dendritic cells pulsed with hepatitis B surface antigen-loaded elastic liposomes. *Vaccine,* 25, 6939-6944.

Mishra, D.; Mishra, P.K.; Dubey, V.; Nahar, M.; Dabadghao, S.; Jain, N.K. (2008). Systemic and mucosal immune response induced by transcutaneous immunization using Hepatitis B surface antigen-loaded modified liposomes. *Eur. J. Pharm. Sci.*, 33, 424-433.

Nossal, J.V. (2000). The global alliance for vaccines and immunization-a millennial challenge. *Nat. Immunol.,* 1, 5-8.

Paliwal, R.; Paliwal, S.R.; Vyas, S.P. (2010). Advances in effective vaccine development against hepatitis B: focus on mucosal immunization strategies. *Therapeutic Delivery*, 1, 3, 397-410.

Pandey, R.S.; Dixit, V.K. (2010). Evaluation of ISCOM vaccines for mucosal immunization against hepatitis B. *J. Drug Target,* 18, 282-291.

Pandey, R.S.; Dixit, V.K. (2009). Evaluation of ISCOMs for immunization against hepatitis B. *Curr. Pharm. Biotechnol.,* 10, 709-716.

Papaevangelou, G. (1998). Current combined vaccines with hepatitis B. *Vaccine*, 16, S69-72.

Partidos, C.D. (2000). Intranasal vaccines: forthcoming challenges. *Pharm. Sci. Technol.* Today, 3, 273-280.

Paul, A.; Cevc, G.; Bachhawat, B.K. (1998). Transdermal immunisation with an integral membrane component, gap junction protein, by means of ultradeformable drug carriers, transfersomes. *Vaccine*, 16, 188-195.

Pawar, D.; Goyal, A.K.; Mangal, S.; *et al.* (2010) Evaluation of Mucoadhesive PLGA Microparticles for Nasal Immunization. *AAPS J.*, 12, 130-137.

Perrie, Y.; Frederik, P.M.; Gregoriadis, G. (2001). Liposome-mediated DNA vaccination: the effect of vesicle composition. *Vaccine,* 19, 3301-3310.

Saini, V.; Sahoo, M.K.; Murthy, P.K.; Kohli, D. (2009). Polymeric lamellar substrate particles as carrier adjuvant for recombinant hepatitis B surface antigen vaccine. *Vaccine*. 27, 2372-2378.

Sanyal, G.; Shi, L. (2009). A review of multiple approaches towards an improved hepatitis B vaccine. *Expert Opin. Ther. Pat.*, 19, 59-72.

Shi, L.; Caulfield, M.J.; Chern, R.T.; Wilson, R.A.; Sanyal, G.; Volkin, D.B. (2002). Pharmaceutical and immunological evaluation of a single-shot hepatitis B vaccine formulated with PLGA microspheres. *J. Pharm. Sci.,* 91, 1019-1035.

Shukla, A.; Katare, O.P.; Singh, B.; Vyas, S.P. (2010). M-cell targeted delivery of recombinant hepatitis B surface antigen using cholera toxin B subunit conjugated bilosomes. *Int. J. Pharm.,* 385, 47-52.

Shukla, A.; Khatri, K.; Gupta, P.N.; Goyal, A.K.; Mehta, A.; Vyas, S.P. (2008). Oral immunization against hepatitis B using bile salt stabilized vesicles (bilosomes). *J. Pharm. Pharm. Sci.,* 11, 59-66.

Simerska, P.; Moyle, P.M.; Olive, C.; Toth, I. (2009). Oral vaccine delivery--new strategies and technologies. *Curr. Drug Deliv.*, 6, 347-358.

Slutter; B.; Hagenaars, N.; Jiskoot, W. (2008). Rational design of nasal vaccines. *J. Drug Target*, 16, 1-17.

Thoelen, S.; De Clercq, N.; Tornieporth, N. (2001). A prophylactic hepatitis B vaccine with a novel adjuvant system. *Vaccine*, 19, 2400-2403.

Tiollais, P.; Pourcel, C.; Dejean, A. (1985). The hepatitis B virus. *Nature*, 317, 489–495.

Tiwari, S.; Verma, S.K.; Agrawal, G.P.; Vyas, S.P. (2011). Viral protein complexed liposomes for intranasal delivery of hepatitis B surface antigen. *Int. J. Pharm.*, 413, 211-219.

Tiwari, S.; Vyas, S.P. (2011). Novel approaches to oral immunization for hepatitis B. *Curr. Infect. Dis. Rep.* 2011, 13, 4-12.

Vyas, S.P.; Gupta, P.N. (2007). Implication of nanoparticles/microparticles in mucosal vaccine delivery. *Expert Rev. Vaccines*, 6, 401-418.

Vyas, S.P.; Singh, R.P.; Jain, S.; *et al.* (2005). Non-ionic surfactant based vesicles (niosomes) for non-invasive topical genetic immunization against hepatitis B. *Int. J. Pharm.,* 296, 80-86.

Wang, J.; Hu, J. H.; Li, F.Q.; *et al.* (2007). Strong cellular and humoral immune responses induced by transcutaneous immunization with HBsAg DNA-cationic deformable liposome complex. *Exp. Dermatol.,* 16, 724-729.

Watson, D.S.; Endsley, A.N.; Huang, L. (2012). Design considerations for liposomal vaccines: influence of formulation parameters on antibody and cell-mediated immune responses to liposome associated antigens. *Vaccine*, 30, 2256-2272.

Reviewed by: Dr. K. C. Gupta, Director, Indian Institute of Toxicological Research, Lucknow, India

In: Hepatitis B: New Research
Editors: J. T. Cox and D. I. Owen
ISBN 978-1-62081-846-6

Chapter IV

Management of Chronic Hepatitis B

Walid S. Ayoub [*] ***and Channa R. Jayasekera*** [2]
[1]Department of Gastroenterology and Hepatology, Stanford University, US
[2]Department of Internal Medicine, Stanford University, California, US

Introduction

At least two billion people worldwide are estimated to have exposure to hepatitis B infection. Forty-five percent of these exposures occur in areas of high endemicity such as Central and South-East Asia, sub-Saharan Africa, and the Amazon Basin, where population prevalence of hepatitis B is greater than 8% and lifetime risk of infection – occurring primarily during childhood – is greater than 60%. A further 43% of exposures occur in areas with 2-7% prevalence, where lifetime risk ranges between 20 and 60%. In contrast, areas of low prevalence, which include the United States, Western Europe, Australia, and parts of South America, account for the remaining 12% of exposures, where prevalence is less than 2%, with exposures occurring largely in adulthood [1].

Recent advances in genotyping have helped develop a more nuanced understanding of the distribution of hepatitis B. At least ten hepatitis B

[*] Correspondent author: Walid Ayoub, MD. wayoub@stanford.edu

genotypes, A-J, as well some subtypes have been identified. Genotypes A, D and E account for a large majority of isolates in sub-Saharan Africa and Central Asia. Genotypes B and C dominate South-East Asia while genotypes A and F are prevalent in the Amazon Basin [2].

Chronic hepatitis B (CHB) carries a significant global burden. It accounts for 30% of cases of cirrhosis, 53% of cases of hepatocellular carcinoma and 620,000 yearly deaths worldwide [3]. Of the 350 million people chronically infected worldwide, a large majority resides in countries of high prevalence.

In the United States, the prevalence of CHB is estimated to range between 1.4 to 2 million, and is influenced by factors such as immigration of chronically infected persons from high prevalence areas, perinatal transmission, transmission among contacts, and high-risk behaviors [1, 4, 5].

Vaccination is among the most important and cost-effective interventions in eradicating or controlling hepatitis B. However, despite a highly effective and safe vaccine being available since 1982, global coverage of complete vaccination is only 60%, notably with the lowest coverage in regions of highest endemicity [6]. Several countries with high endemicity have had dramatic reductions in CHB prevalence since the institution of population-wide immunization. In China for instance, where birth-dose vaccination covers more than 80% of newborns, the prevalence of CHB in children under five years is now estimated to be less than 1%, compared with a population prevalence of approximately 10% [7]. In the United States where universal vaccination was instituted in 1991, there has been a 79% reduction in CHB prevalence in children six to 19 years, from 1.9% to 0.6% [8].

Given that global vaccination programs still fall short of universal coverage, and that vaccination has no impact on the clinical course of CHB, anti-viral therapy for individuals with CHB itself is an area of intensive research. The goal of anti-viral therapy is to reduce or eliminate the risk of progression of CHB to cirrhosis, hepatic decompensation, and hepatocellular carcinoma.

Natural History of Hepatitis B

Hepatitis B virus is consistently present in blood, semen, saliva, and to variable extents in milk, vaginal and menstrual secretions, and amniotic fluid of infected individuals. The likelihood of infection is greatest with direct inoculation of blood, such as through transfusion of contaminated blood products and percutaneous introduction by contaminated needles. Vertical transmission from mother to child and prolonged non-sexual interactions with household contacts account for the majority of infections in areas of high endemicity. Sexual transmission is however estimated to be the most common means of transmission in the United States, accounting for almost 50% of infections [9].

Infection with hepatitis B leads to either complete clearance of the virus or development of a chronic state. The likelihood of clearance is highly contingent upon the age at infection, ranging from less than 10% of neonatal or early childhood infections to greater than 95% of adult infections [10].

Acute infection is characterized by elevated serum alanine aminotransferase (ALT), and the presence of hepatitis B surface antigen (HBsAg), anti-hepatitis B core IgM (anti-HBc), and the marker of viral replication, hepatitis B e antigen (HBeAg). However, fewer than 30% of individuals develop obvious physical manifestations of acute infection such as jaundice [11].

Progression of CHB is classically divided into four phases: immune tolerance, immune clearance, seroconversion to inactive carrier, and reactivation. The hallmarks of the immune tolerance phase are high viral replication within the hepatocytes as detected by the presence of HBeAg, elevated serum HBV DNA and normal ALT level. Histologically, there is little if any liver inflammation or fibrosis. Thus, existing data suggest that the immune tolerance phase typically portends a favorable prognosis over at least a decade [12].

The immune clearance phase is marked by persistent HBe antigenemia, high serum HBV DNA as well as fluctuating elevations in ALT due to immune-mediated destruction of infected hepatocytes. Histologically, this phase is marked by inflammation and varying degrees of fibrosis.

Seroconversion, which occurs at a rate of 10-20% per year in untreated individuals, is marked by the development of antibodies to HBeAg (anti-HBe) and eventual clearance of the HBeAg. Seroconversion transitions individuals into the inactive carrier phase of disease, which is characterized by little or no viral replication activity and thereby undetectable serum HBV DNA , normal ALT, and minimal fibrosis on histology [12, 13]. A small percentage of individuals in the inactive phase may also develop antibodies to HBsAg (anti-HBs), though low level viremia persists with DNA detectable by polymerase chain reaction and on liver biopsy [13].

The reactivation phase may be either spontaneous or triggered by immunosuppression, characterized by precore or core promoter mutant HBV viruses that suppress the expression of HBeAg. Less commonly, reactivation can be due to resurgence of the wild type virus [12, 13]. Reactivation is therefore classically manifested by an undetectable HBeAg, but persistently high serum HBV DNA, elevated ALT level, as well as histological evidence of significant inflammation and fibrosis.

Finally, the role of HBV genotype in the progression of disease remains under investigation. For instance, data from comparative studies suggest that patients with CHB genotypes A and B progress to seroconversion sooner than patients with CHB genotype D and C. In addition, genotypes A1, C, B2-B5, and F1 CHB is associated with more serious complications from chronic liver disease than genotypes A2, B1, and B6 CHB [2].

Chronic Hepatitis B Therapies

The primary goal of antiviral therapy is to retard the progression of CHB to cirrhosis, hepatocellular carcinoma, and liver failure. Several viral, host, and environmental factors are associated with disease progression, including persistently high serum HBV DNA, persistently detectable HBeAg, presence of core promoter mutations, male gender, older age, hepatitis exacerbations, persistently elevated ALT, the presence of cirrhosis, diabetes, or concurrent hepatitis C, hepatitis D, or HIV, and alcohol or tobacco abuse [12]. Among these, serum HBV DNA, which corresponds to viral replication, remains the strongest known correlate of progression. This was evidenced by two large prospective studies with over 3500 subjects where elevated serum HBV DNA was found to be the strongest predictor of progression to both cirrhosis and hepatocellular carcinoma, independent of HBeAg status and serum ALT levels [14, 15]. Consequently, HBV DNA level is the key determinants of initiating therapy, and its suppression is one of the key end-points of treatment.

Seven agents are now approved by the United States Food and Drug Administration for treatment of CHB. These include two interferons and five oral agents.

The two interferons, interferon alfa-2b (IFN) and pegylated interferon alfa-2a (PegIFN), possess both anti-viral and immunomodulatory properties. The oral agents consist of five nucleos(t)ide analogues: lamivudine, adefovir dipivoxil, entecavir, telbivudine, and tenofovir disproxil fumarate. Unlike the interferons, the oral agents have only anti-viral properties.

Interferon

Interferon alfa-2b (IFN) has been shown in multiple studies to be associated with suppressed viral replication, decreased incidence of decompensation and hepatocellular carcinoma, and increased survival during long-term follow up. A large meta-analysis of 24 randomized controlled trials and 12 cohort studies of HBeAg-positive individuals, showed IFN to be superior to placebo in inducing HBV DNA suppression (NNT = 4.3), HBeAg clearance (NNT = 4.1), and HBsAg clearance (NNT = 17.1) [16]. Follow-up of patients treated with IFN have shown persistent clearance of HBsAg, improved liver histology, lower rates of hepatocellular carcinoma, and increased absolute survival and complication-free survival in both HBeAg positive and negative individuals [17, 18]. However, given the need for daily or three-times weekly injections, a less favorable side-effect profile, and possibly inferior efficacy, IFN has now been largely replaced by once-weekly pegylated IFN alfa-2a (PegIFN).

In HBeAg-positive CHB, 48-52 weeks of PegIFN monotherapy have been shown to result in 32-36% clearance of HBeAg, 7-14% suppression of HBV DNA below 400 copies/ml, and 4-6% emergence of anti-HBs, when assessed 24 weeks after therapy [19, 20]. In a mean three-year follow up, 81% of individuals who initially cleared HBeAg were found to have a sustained response [21]. In HBeAg-negative CHB, a 12-month course of PegIFN resulted in 19% of subjects achieving serum HBV DNA below 400 copies/ml at 6 months [22]. In a three-year follow up, 15% of individuals continued to have sustained suppression of HBV DNA below 400 copies/ml, and 8% of patients had HBsAg loss. The addition of lamivudine to PEG-IFN did not synergize serocoversion in either HBeAg positive or HBeAg negative subjects. It led to a more rapid suppression of HBV DNA during and immediately after treatment in addition to lower rate of emergence of viral resistance. [19-22].

The impact of hepatitis B genotypes on interferon response was reflected in an analysis of 542 HBeAg-positive subjects treated with PegIFN for 48 weeks. The best responses to interferon were seen in genotype A with high ALT or low HBV DNA, and genotypes B and C with high ALT and low HBV DNA. Genotype D was associated with the poorest sustained responses [23]. The analysis also led to the development of the interferon HBV treatment index (www.liver-gi.nl/peg-ifn). This treatment index offers a predicted probability of achieving a sustained response in interferon-naïve patients based on the HBV genotype (A-D), levels of ALT and HBV DNA, gender, and age.

The rate of decline of HBsAg has also been linked to the likelihood of achieving sustained virological response with interferon based therapy. HBeAg-positive patients who do not demonstrate a decline in serum HBsAg in the first 12 weeks of therapy have been shown to be significantly less likely to achieve sustained response or loss of HBsAg [24]. In comparison, sustained response in HBeAg-negative subjects appears to be associated with a more vigorous decline in HBsAg titer, or a lower HBsAg titer at 12 weeks of therapy [25].

Nucleos(t)ide Analogues

A central mechanism in the pathogenesis of hepatitis B is translation of the HBV DNA genome into pre-genomic viral RNA, which in-turn through reverse transcription, serves as the template for synthesis of viral DNA within hepatocytes. The primary mechanism of action of currently approved nucleos(t)ide analogues is the inhibition of this reverse transcription of HBV pre-genomic RNA. To date, five nucleos(t)ide analogues belonging to three classes have been approved for use by the United States Food and Drug Administration, namely, lamivudine and telbivudine (L-nucleosides), adefovir dipivoxil and tenfovir (acyclic nucleosides), and entecavir (deoxyguanosine analogue).

Lamivudine

Lamivudine, approved for use in the United States since 1998, has been shown to be beneficial in inducing HBV DNA suppression, ALT normalization, and in retarding histological change irrespective of HBeAg status. In addition, it has been shown to induce HBeAg seroconversion in HbeAg positive individuals. In early studies of HBeAg-positive subjects, one-year therapy with lamivudine compared with placebo was associated with 44% versus 16% suppression of HBV DNA to undetectable levels, 52% versus 23% histologic response, and 32% versus 11% loss of HBeAg [26]. The HBeAg seroconversion rate increased to 35-65% after 5 years of therapy. The increased seroconversion rate was associated with prolonged duration of therapy and elevated pre-treatment ALT levels, particularly when ALT is over 5-times the upper limit of normal [27]. Treatment with lamivudine is also associated with lower rates of hepatic fibrosis and hepatocellular carcinoma. In a study of over 600 subjects with advanced fibrosis, rates of hepatic decompensation, hepatic encephalopathy, hepatocellular carcinoma, spontaneous bacterial peritonitis, variceal bleeding, and death due to liver disease were significantly lower in those treated with lamivudine, compared to placebo (7.8% versus 17.7%) over a median duration of 32 months. Furthermore, subjects in the lamivudine treatment arm were also less likely to have an increase in Child-Pugh score (3.4% vs. 8.8%) and had lower rates of hepatocellular carcinoma (3.9% versus 7.4%) [28].

In HBeAg-positive individuals, lamivudine can be stopped in the setting of HBeAg seroconversion and after a period of consolidation with a low risk for hepatitis B relapse. In HBeAg-negative individuals, lamivudine therapy is indefinite since the risk of relapse is high after stopping therapy.

The durability of HBV DNA suppression with lamivudine, irrespective of HBeAg status, is lower than interferon therapy, ranging between 50-80% in HBeAg-positive individuals, and 20-25% in HBeAg-negative individuals [19-22]. Moreover, development of lamivudine resistance with the emergence of mutations in the YMDD motif of the polymerase gene has been known to occur in as few as six months of therapy, and increase concomitantly with duration of treatment [29]. Consequently, five years of therapy can lead to a 65-70% rate of resistance [30]. The availability of other antiviral agents with better resistance profiles has resulted in significant decrease in the use of lamivudine in the United States.

Adefovir Dipivoxil

Adefovir, approved in 2002, is active against both wild-type and lamivudine-resistant HBV. In a trial of one-year 10mg daily adefovir therapy versus placebo in HBeAg-positive subjects, the adefovir treatment arm had better rates of HBeAg seroconversion (12% versus 6%), histological improvement (53% versus 25%), reduction in serum HBV DNA to undetectable levels (21% versus 0%), and ALT normalization (48% versus 16%) [31]. Furthermore, the seroconversion has been reported to be durable for at least three years in over 90% of the same subjects [32]. In HBeAg-negative subjects, 1 year of adefovir therapy resulted in HBV DNA suppression and ALT normalization in 51% and 72% of patients when compared to 0% and 29% in subjects administered placebo [33]. Treatment-naïve HBeAg-negative patients treated for 192 to 240 weeks with adefovir have shown significant improvement in necroinflammation (83%), fibrosis (73%), suppression of serum HBV DNA below 1000 copies/ml (67%), and in normalization of ALT (69%) [34]. The development of resistance to adefovir correlates with duration of exposure, with rates of 3%, 8%, 18%, 22%, and 30% at 1, 2, 3, 4, and 5 years of therapy, respectively [33]. Moreover, the use of adefovir has been declining due to data suggesting superior outcomes with the structurally similar, newer nucleotide analogue, tenofovir.

Entecavir

Entecavir is a potent HBV polymerase inhibitor approved for use in the United States in 2005. In HBeAg-positive subjects, 52 weeks of entecavir therapy has been shown to be more efficacious than lamivudine therapy in suppressing HBV DNA below 400 copies/ml (67% versus 36%), histological improvement (72% versus 62%), and normalization of ALT (78% versus 70%) [35]. However, this study did not show a statistically significant different rate of serocoversion in HBeAg-positive subjects treated with either entecavir or lamivudine (21% versus 18%). Extending entecavir therapy to 96 and 192 weeks in partial responders was shown to result in even higher rates of HBV DNA suppression compared to lamivudine (91% and 74%), ALT normalization (86% and 79%), and seroconversion (31% and an additional 16%) respectively [36, 37]. Entecavir has also been shown to be superior to lamivudine in HBeAg-negative subjects. A 48 week course of entecavir versus lamivudine demonstrated HBV DNA suppression below 400 copies/ml in 90% versus 72%, histological improvement in 70% versus 61%, and normalization of ALT in 78% versus 71% of subjects [38]. Moreover, entecavir when compared with adefovir in HBeAg-positive subjects, achieved higher rates of viral suppression at 48 weeks, HBV clearance (58% versus 19%), and ALT normalization (76% versus 63%). However the rates of HBeAg loss and HBeAg seroconversion were comparable [39]. Finally, both HBeAg-positive and HBeAg-negative subjects, including those with cirrhosis, were found to have improved hepatic fibrosis scores as well as histological improvement on biopsy compared to their baselines after treated six years of therapy [40].

Entecavir has a high genetic barrier to resistance, with resistance requiring at least three mutations, resulting in a 0.8% incidence of resistance with virologic breakthrough at five years of therapy in nucleoside-naïve subjects [41]. This rate is expectedly higher in subjects with documented nucleoside-resistance. Entecavir resistance was encountered in almost 40% of subjects with documented lamivudine resistance at four years of therapy [42].

Telbivudine

Approved for use in the United States in 2006, telbivudine is one of the newer nucleosides available for treatment of CHB. Its superiority over lamivudine among both HBeAg-negative and positive disease was demonstrated in a phase III trial with over 1300 subjects [43]. Telbivudine leads to significantly better suppression than lamivudine of HBV DNA after 12 weeks of therapy in HBeAg-positive subjects (5.71 $\log_{10}$ versus 5.42$\log_{10}$) and in HBeAg-negative subjects (4.36$\log_{10}$ versus 4.08$\log_{10}$). 52 weeks of therapy of telbivudine in HBeAg-positive subjects resulted in better therapeutic response, described as HBV DNA suppression below 5 $\log_{10}$ copies/ml along with HBeAg loss, or normalization of ALT (75.3% versus 67%) when compared with lamivudine. Additionally, telbivudine therapy led to better histological improvement (64.7% versus 56.3%). In HBeAg-negative subjects, the rates of response were non-inferior to those treated with lamivudine. Rates of resistance at 52 weeks were also lower in the telbividuine group for both HBeAg-positive and negative individuals, compared to the lamivudine group (5.0% and 2.3% versus 11% and 10.7%, respectively).

These findings were further validated after two years of treatment in the GLOBE trial. Compared to lamivudine, telbivudine therapy led to better therapeutic response in HBeAg-positive subjects (63% versus 48%) and in HBeAg-negative subjects (78% versus 66%). Undetectable HBV DNA was reported in 55.6% versus 38.5% of HBeAg-positive subjects, and 82% versus 56.7% of HBeAg-negative subjects [44]. Extending telbivudine therapy up to three years resulted in 77% and 37% of HBeAg-positive subjects demonstrating undetectable HBV DNA and HBeAg seroconversion, respectively. Furthermore, at three years, 84% of subjects sustained the HBeAg seroconversion achieved during two years of therapy. In HBeAg-negative subjects, the complete suppression of HBV and normalization of ALT were in 85% and 83% of subjects respectively. Resistance rates at two and three years were reported as 25.1% and 11.3% in HBeAg-positive subjects and 10.8% and 6.5% in HBeAg-negative subjects [43, 45].

In HBeAg-positive subjects, telbivudine was also found to be superior to lamivudine in suppressing HBV DNA by 24 weeks of therapy (39% versus 12%). At 52 weeks, this suppression to undetectable limits was 60% versus

40%. The telbivudine treated arm also had higher seroconversion rates at the end of treatment, 28% versus 19% [46]. However, the use of telbivudine has been limited by its intermediate barrier to resistance.

Tenofovir

Tenofovir was approved for therapy of CHB in the United States in 2008. While structurally similar to adefovir, tenofovir has been shown to have superior outcomes in terms of HBV DNA suppression, HBeAg seroconversion, and normalization of ALT. Tenofovir also has an unmatched resistance profile, with no reported cases of resistance in CHB patients who are HIV negative [47].

In a trial that evaluated tenofovir versus adefovir, tenofovir was found to result in markedly better rates of HBV DNA suppression to less than 400 copies/ml at 48 weeks of therapy (76% versus 13%) in HBeAg-positive subjects. Furthermore, this group also had better outcomes in normalization of ALT (68% versus 54%), comparable rates of HBeAg seroconversion (21% versus 18%), and histological improvement (74% versus 68%). Three percent of subjects treated with tenofovir were also found to lose HBsAg at the end of 48 weeks. Among HBeAg-negative subjects in this study, the rate of HBV DNA suppression to less than 400 copies/ml was 93% in the tenofovir arm, versus 63% in those who received adefovir. Overall, 66% of HBeAg-positive subjects and 71% of HBeAg-negative subjects treated with tenofovir demonstrated viral suppression and histologic improvement compared with 12% and 49% treated with adefovir, respectively [48].

Extending tenofovir therapy to 5 years resulted in continuous sustained[d] viral suppression. 97% of HBeAg-positive and 99% of HBeAg-negative subjects demonstrated HBV viral suppression defined as HBV DNA less than 400 copies/ml based on on-treatment analysis. Five years of tenofovir therapy was also associated with histological improvement and ALT normalization in 88% and 73% of HBeAg-positive subjects and 87% and 85% of HBeAg-negative subjects respectively. Of 94 subjects who were cirrhotic at baseline, 74% demonstrated at least a 2-point reduction in their Ishak fibrosis score, attesting to regression of cirrhosis in these subjects. Loss of HBsAg was seen in 10% of HBeAg-positive subjects and 0.3% of HBeAg-negative subjects. Moreover, none of the 490 subjects developed resistance to tenofovir after five years of ongoing therapy [49].

Table 1. Treatment efficacy with oral nucleos(t)ides at one year (Studies are not head to head comparisions) [47]

	Lamivudine [43]	Adefovir [31,33]	Telbivudine [43]	Entecavir [35,38]	Tenofovir [48]
HBeAg-Positive					
Undetectable HBV DNA	60%	48%	77%	68%	68%
HBeAg seroconversion	36%	21%	60%	67%	76%
ALT normalization	18%	12%	21%	21%	21%
HBeAg-Negative					
Undetectable HBV DNA	71%	72%	74%	74%	76%
ALT normalization	72%	51%	88%	88%	93%

Safety

Both IFN and PegIFN are associated with influenza-type symptoms in a significant proportion of patients. Association of interferon with depression, irritability, and suicidal ideations make it necessary to screen patients for neuropsychiatric disease prior to initiation of therapy. Other common adverse effects include anorexia, autoimmune disease flares, thyroid dysfunction, myelosuppression, psoriasis exacerbation and hepatitis flares. Furthermore, interferons are contraindicated in patients with decompensated cirrhosis due to the risks of sepsis and liver failure [12, 50].

Nucleos(t)ide analogues are generally well tolerated during the treatment of CHB. As a class, they carry the potential risk of causing lactic acidosis. Adefovir has been associated with an approximately 3-6% risk of proximal renal tubular dysfunction as manifested by acute or chronic renal insufficiency, and possibly Fanconi syndrome [51, 52]. Nephrotoxicity of tenofovir in monoinfected hepatitis B patients is controversial. To date, there has been no reported significant renal dysfunction in the tenofovir registration trials of hepatitis B monoinfected patients. Decreased bone density and osteomalacia have been reported with the use of tenofovir in patients co-infected with HBV and HIV but have not been seen in moninfected patients with hepatitis B so far. Lactic acidosis has been reported in six patients with cirrhosis with Model for End-Stage Liver Disease (MELD) scores greater or equal to 20 on entecavir therapy [53]. Finally, peripheral neuropathy, reversible symptomatic myopathy and asymptomatic elevations of creatine kinase greater than seven-times upper limit of normal have also been reported with the use of telbivudine [44].

Resistance

Nucleos(t)ide analogue resistance is the result of adaptive HBV polymerase gene mutations, occurring under selection pressure during antiviral therapy [54]. Resistance is a common phenomenon and is the most significant limitation to their use.

The initial manifestation of resistance is virologic breakthrough, defined as an increase in HBV DNA by greater than 1 log_{10} (10-fold) from its nadir, or, in patients who have previously had undetectable HBV DNA, a re-detection of HBV DNA at a level at least 10-fold the lower limit of detectability. Virologic breakthrough is confirmed when the HBV DNA elevation is persistent over a 1-3 month period at the same or higher level.

Biochemical breakthrough, defined as a rise in ALT levels in patients with previously normal ALT, may follow virologic breakthrough. Other downstream manifestations can include hepatitis flares or liver failure. The consequent emergence of clinical symptoms is termed clinical breakthrough [12, 30].

The reported emergence of resistance however varies considerably between drugs and is often directly proportional to the duration of their use (Figure 1). In addition, emergence of resistance is related to drug potency (inadequate viral suppression), patient adherence, viral replication fitness, mechanism of drug action, and cross-resistance patterns between drugs to which the patient has been exposed [55].

This last factor explains the high rates of resistance seen in patients who have previously failed therapy. It is therefore crucial to choose an agent with a high genetic barrier to mutation as a first line therapy. Moreover, monitoring for adequate viral suppression early on in treatment at 12 and 24 weeks of therapy is important to minimizing risk of resistance since the selection of mutants is a function of suboptimal viral suppression [57].

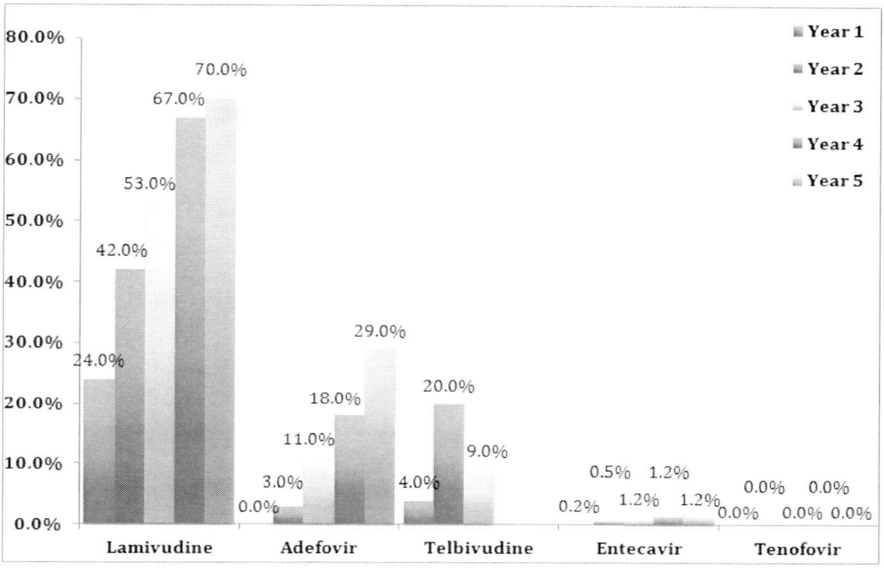

Figure 1. Reported hepatitis B viral resistance with the use of oral nucleos(t)ides.

The genetic barrier to resistance is lowest in lamivudine, intermediate in adefovir and telbivudine, and highest in entecavir and tenofovir. Developing resistance to lamivudine increases the risk of developing mutations to the other nucleosides (telbivudine and entacavir). Similarly, developing resistance to adefovir has the theoretical risk of causing resistance to tenofovir (Table 2).

Table 2. Resistance-Conferring HBV Polymerase Gene Mutations

Genetic Barrier	Nucleos(t)ide Analogue	HBV Polymerase Gene Mutations
Low	Lamivudine	rtA181T/V, rtM204V/I/S
Intermediate	Adefovir	rtA181T/V, rtN236T, rtI233V
	Telbivudine	rtM204I, rtA181T/V, rtL229W/V
High	Entecavir	rtM204V/I + rtL180M ± rtL169 ± rtS184G ± rtS2021 ± rtM250V
	Tenofovir	?rt181T/V, ?rtN236T

Table 3. Management of Chronic hepatitis B according to the treatment guidelines

		HBV DNA (IU/ml)	Other	Treatment Strategy
HBeAg-Positive Chronic Hepatitis B	US Algorithm [57]	>20,000	ALT > ULN	Treat
		>20,000	ALT Normal	Consider liver biopsy if age > 35 years
		>2000	Compensated Cirrhosis	Treat. Consider treatment if HBV DNA <2000 IU/ml
		Any	Decompensated Cirrhosis	Treat
	AASLD [58]	>20,000	ALT ≤2 x ULN	Observe Age >40 or ALT persistently 1-2 x ULN or family history of HCC: Consider biopsy. Treat if biopsy shows significant histological disease.
		>2000	ALT >2 x ULN	Treat if no spontaneous HBeAg loss in 3-6 months Compensated: Treat. Consider liver biopsy prior to treatment. Decompensated: Treat
		Detectable	Cirrhosis	Compensated + HBV DNA >2000 IU/ml: Treat Compensated + HBV DNA <2000 IU/ml: Consider treatment if elevated ALT Decompensated: Treat + refer for transplant
		Undetectable	Cirrhosis	Compensated: Observe Decompensated: Refer for transplant
	EASL [59]	>2000	And/or ALT > ULN	Consider liver biopsy. Treat if biopsy shows significant histological disease.
		Detectable	Cirrhosis	Compensated: Treat Decompensated: Treat
	APASL [60]	>20,000	ALT >5 x ULN	Treat
		>20,000	ALT 2 to 5 x ULN	ALT elevation persistent for 3-6 months: Treat Decompensated: Treat
		>20,000	ALT <2 x ULN	Perform liver biopsy. Treat if moderate/severe inflammation or fibrosis.

		HBV DNA (IU/ml)	Other	Treatment Strategy
HBeAg-Negative Chronic Hepatitis B	US Algorithm[57]	>2000	ALT > ULN	Treat
		>2000	ALT Normal	Consider liver biopsy if age > 35 years
		HBV DNA (IU/ml)	Other	Treatment Strategy
		>2000	CompensatedCirrhosis	Treat. Consider treatment if HBV DNA <2000 IU/ml
		Any	Decompensated Cirrhosis	Treat
	AASLD[58]	>2,000	ALT >2 x ULN	Treat
		>2000	ALT 1 to >2 x ULN	Consider biopsy. Treat if biopsy shows significant histological disease.
		≤2000	ALT ≤ ULN	Observe
		Detectable	Cirrhosis	Compensated + HBV DNA >2000 IU/ml: Treat Compensated + HBV DNA <2000 IU/ml: Consider treatment if elevated ALT Decompensated: Treat and refer for transplant
		Undetectable	Cirrhosis	Compensated: Observe Decompensated: Refer for transplant
	EASL[59]	>2000	ALT > ULN	Consider liver biopsy. Treat if biopsy shows significant histological disease.
		Detectable	Cirrhosis	Compensated: Treat Decompensated: Treat
	APASL[60]	>2000	ALT >2 x ULN	ALT elevation persistent for 3-6 months: Treat
		>2000	ALT <2 x ULN	Perform liver biopsy. Treat if moderate/severe inflammation or fibrosis
		>2000	Cirrhosis	Treat
		Any	Decompensated Cirrhosis	Treat

Treatment Guidelines

Several major societies including the American Association for the Study of the Liver (AASLD), European Association Study of the Liver (EASL), and the Asian Pacific Association for the Study of the Liver (APASL), as well as other expert consensus panels have issued recommended guidelines for initiation of treatment of chronic hepatitis B (Table 3).

Current guidelines emphasize the importance of using an agent with a high genetic barrier such as entecavir, tenofovir or PegIFN, as a first line agent. Superior efficacy of combination therapy has not borne out in trials, though this strategy is sometimes employed in special situations such as patients with multiple drug resistance or co-infection with HIV [56].

Conclusion

Despite the introduction of drugs with high genetic barriers, the complete eradication of hepatitis B remains challenging. Even with optimal viral suppression, patients remain at risk of developing hepatocellular carcinoma in particular, and to some extent, cirrhosis and hepatic decompensation. Moreover, the presence of intracellular covalently closed circular HBV DNA within hepatocytes allows for potential reactivation of disease in case of discontinuation of therapy or immunosuppression. Given that viral rebound is often seen after discontinuation of therapy, prolonged if not lifelong therapy is often necessary.

Universal hepatitis B vaccination is by far the most cost-effective and definitive preventative strategy for CHB. However, despite increasing global vaccination coverage, the eradication of CHB will be elusive for the foreseeable future, making research on CHB therapeutics, their initiation guidelines, and therapeutic end-points imperative.

References

[1] McHugh JA, Cullison S, Apuzzio J, Block JM, Cohen C, Leong SL, Longon WT, NcNellis RJ, Neubauer RL, Perrillo R, Squires R, Tarrant D, McMahon BJ. 2011. Chronic hepatitis B infection: A workshop

consensus statement and algorithm. *Journal of Family Practice* 60(9), E1-8.

[2] Tanwar S, Dusheiko G. 2012. Is there any value to hepatitis B virus genotype analysis? *Current Gastroenterology Reports* 14, 17-46.

[3] Te HS, Jensen DM. 2010. Epidemiology of hepatitis B and C viruses: A global overview. *Clinical Liver Diseases* 14, 1-21.

[4] Centers for Disease Control and Prevention. Disease burden from hepatitis A, B and C. Available at: http://www.cdc.gov/hepatitis/Statistics/index.htm. Accessed December 18, 2011.

[5] Cohen C, Evans AA, Longon WT, Block JM, Contin M, Block T. 2008. Underestimation of chronic hepatitis B virus infection in the United States of America. *Journal of Viral Hepatology* 46, 1034-40.

[6] Zanetti AR, Van Damme P, Shouval D. 2008. The global impact of vaccination against hepatitis B: A historical overview. *Vaccine* 26, 6266-6273.

[7] WHO, UNICEF, World Bank. 2009. State of the world's vaccines and immunization. 3rd ed. Geneva, World Health Organization.

[8] Wasley A, Kruszon-Moran D, Kuhnert W, Simard EP, Finelli L, McQuillan G, Bell B. 2010. The prevalence of hepatitis B virus infection in the United States in the era of vaccination. *Journal of Infectious Diseases* 202(2), 192-201.

[9] Centers for Disease Control and Prevention. 2004. Incidence of acute hepatitis B – United States, 1990-2002. *Morbidity and Mortality Weekly Report*, 52(51-52), 1252-1254.

[10] Yim HJ, Lok AS. 2006. Natural history of chronic hepatitis B virus infection: what we knew in 1981 and what we know in 2005. *Hepatology* 43(2), Supplement 1, S173-181.

[11] McMahon BJ, Alward WL, Hall DB, Heyward WL, Bender TR, Francis DP, Maynard JE. 1985. Acute hepatitis B virus infection: relation of age to the clinical expression of disease and subsequent development of the carrier state. *Journal of Infectious Disease* 151(4), 599-503.

[12] Kwon H, Lok AS. 2011. Hepatitis B therapy. *Nature Reviews Gastroenterology and Hepatology* 8(5), 275-84.

[13] Fattovich G, Bortolotti F, Donato F. 2008. Natural history of chronic hepatitis B: Special emphasis on disease progression and prognostic factors. *Journal of Hepatology* 48, 335-352.

[14] Iloeje CH, Yang H-I, Su J, Jen C-L, You S-L, Chen C-J. 2006. Predicting cirrhosis risk based on the level of circulating hepatitis B viral load. *Gastroenterology*, 130, 678-686.

[15] Chen C-J, Yang H-I, Su J, Jen C-L, You S-L, Lu S-N, Hunag G-T, Iloeje UH. 2006. Risk of hepatocellular carcinoma across a biological gradient of serum hepatitis B virus DNA level. *Journal of the American Medical Association*, 295(1), 69-73.

[16] Craxi A, Di Bona D, Camma C. 2003. Interferon-α for HBeAg-positive chronic hepatitis B. *Journal of Hepatology*, 39(S1), 99-105.

[17] van Zonneveld, Honkoop P, Hansen BE, Niesters HG, Darwish Mura S, de Man RA, Schalm SW, Janssen HL. 2004. Long-term follow-up of alpha-interferon treatment of patients with chronic hepatitis B. *Hepatology* 39(3), 804-810.

[18] Papatheodoridis GV, Manesis E, Hadziyannis SJ. 2001. The long-term outcome of interferon-alpha treated and untreated patients with chronic hepatitis B. *Journal of Hepatology*. 34(2), 306-313.

[19] Lau GKK, Piratvisuth T, Luo KX, Marcellin P, Thongsawat S, Cooksley G, Gane E, Fried MW, Chow WC, Paik SW, Chang WY, Berg T, Glisiak R, McCloud P, Pluck N et al. 2005. Peginterferon Alfa-2a, Lamivudine, and the combination for HBeAg-positive chronic hepatitis B. *New England Journal of Medicine*, 352(26), 2682-2695.

[20] Janssen HLA, van Zonneveld M, Senturk H, Zeuzem S, Akarca US, Cakaloglu Y, Simon K, So TMK, Gerken G, de Man RA, Niesters HGM, Zondervan P, Hansen B, Schalm SW et al. 2005. Pegylated interferon alfa-2b alone or in combination with lamivudine for HBeAg-positive chronic hepatitis B: a randomised trial. *Lancet* 365(9454), 123-129.

[21] Buster EH, Flink HJ, Cakaloglu Y, Simon K, Troan J, Tabak F, So TMK, Fienman SV, Mach T, Akarca US, Schutten M, Tielemans W, van Vuuren AJ, Hansen BE, Janssen HL. 2008. Sustained HBeAg and HBsAg loss after long-term follow-up of HBeAg-positive patients treated with peginterferon alpha-2b. *Gastroenterology*, 135(2), 459-467.

[22] Marcellin P, Lau GK, Bonino F, Farci P, Hadziyannis S, Jin R, Lu ZM, Pratvisuth T, Germandis G, Yurdaydin C, Diago M, Gurel S, Lau MY, Button P, Pluck N et a. 2004. Peginterferon alfa-2a alone, lamivudine alone, and the two in combination in patients with chronic hepatitis B. *New England Journal of Medicine*, 351(12), 1206-1217.

[23] Buster EH, Hansen BE, Lau GK, Piratvisuth T, Zeuzem S, Steyerberg EW, Janssen HL. 2002. Factors that predict response of patients with hepatitis B e antigen-positive chronic hepatitis B to peginterferon-alfa. *Gastroenterology*, 137(6), 2002-2009.

[24] Sonneveld MJ, Rijckborst V, Boucher CA, Hansen BE, Janssen HL. 2010. Prediction of sustained response to peginterferon alfa-2b for hepatitis B e antigen-positive chronic hepatitis B using on-treatment hepatitis B surface antigen decline. *Hepatology*, 52(4), 1251-1257.

[25] Rijckborst V, Hansen BE, Cakaloglu Y, Ferenci P, Tabak F, Akdogan M, Simon K, Akarca US, Flisiak R, Verhey E, van Vuuren AJ, Boucher CA, ter Bork MJ, Janssen HL. 2010. Early on-treatment prediction of response in peginterferon alfa-2a for chronic hepatitis B using HBsAg and HBV DNA levels. *Hepatology*, 52(2), 454-461.

[26] Dienstag JL, Schiff ER, Wright TL, Perrillo RP, Hann HW, Goodman Z, Crowther L, Condreay LD, Woessner M, Rubin M, Brown NA. 1999. Lamivudine as initial treatment for chronic hepatitis B in the United States. *New England Journal of Medicine*, 341(17), 1256-1263.

[27] Liaw Y-F. 2003. Results of lamivudine trials in Asia. *Journal of Hepatology*, 39(S1), 111-115.

[28] Liaw Y-F, Sung JJY, Chow WC, Farrell G, Lee C-Z, Yuen H, Tanwandee T, Tao Q-M, Shue K, Keene ON, Dixon JS, Gray F, Sabbat J. 2004. Lamivudine for patients with chronic hepatitis B and advanced liver disease. *New England Journal of Medicine*, 351(15), 1521-1531.

[29] Leung N. 2008. Recent data on treatment of chronic hepatitis B with nucleos(t)ide analogues. *Hepatology International*, 2(2), 163-178.

[30] Ayoub WS, Keeffe EB. 2011. Review article: current antiviral therapy of chronic hepatitis B. *Alimentary Pharmacology and Therapeutics*, 34, 1145-1158.

[31] Marcellin P, Chang TT, Lim SG, Tong MJ, Sievert W, Shiffman ML, Jeffers L, Goodman Z, Wulfsohn MS, Xiong S, Fry J, Brosgart CL. 2003. Adefovir dipivoxil for the treatment of hepatitis B e antigen-positive chronic hepatitis B. *New England Journal of Medicine*, 348(9), 808-816.

[32] Wu IC, Shiffman ML, Tong MJ, Marcellin P, Mondou E, Federick D, Snow-Lampart A, Sorbel J, Rousseau F, Chang TT. Sustained hepatitis B e antigen seroconversion in patients in chronic hepatitis B after adefovir dipivoxil treatment: analysis of precore and basal core promoter mutants. Clinical Infectious Diseases.

[33] Hadziyannis SJ, Tassopoulos NC, Heathcote EJ, Chang TT, Kitis G, Rizzetto M, Marcellin P, Lim SG, Goodman Z, Wilfsohn MS, Xiong S, Fry S, Brosgart CL. 2003. Adefovir dipivoxil for treatment of hepatitis B e antigen-negative chronic hepatitis B. New E*ngland Journal of Medicine*, 348(9), 800-807.

[34] Hadziyannis SJ, Tassopoulos NC, Heathcote EJ, Chang TT, Kitis G, Rizzetto M, Marcellin P, Lim SQ, Goodman Z, Ma J, Brosgart CL, Borroto-Esoda K, Arterburn S, Chuck SL. 2006. Long-term therapy with adefovir dipivoxil for chronic hepatitis B for up to five years. *Gastroenterology*, 131(6), 1743-1751.

[35] Chang TT, Gish RG, de Man R, Gadano A, Sollano J, Chao YC, Lok AS, Han KH, Goodman Z, Zhu J, Cross A, DeHertogh D, Wilber R, Colonno R, Apelian D. 2006. A comparison of entecavir and lamivudine for HBeAg-positive chronic hepatitis B. *New England Journal of Medicine*, 354(10), 1001-1010.

[36] Gish RG, Lok AS, Chang TT, de Man RA, Gadano A, Sollano J, Han KH, Chao YC, Lee SD, Harris M, Yang J, Colonno R, Brett-Smith H. 2007. Entecavir therapy for up to 96 weeks in patients with HBeAg-positive chronic hepatitis B. *Gastroenterology*, 133(5), 1437-1444.

[37] Leung N. 2008. Recent data on treatment of chronic hepatitis B with nucleos(t)ide analogues. *Hepatology International*, 2(2), 163-178.

[38] Lai CL, Shouval D, Lok AS, Chang TT, Cheinquer H, Goodman Z, DeHertogh D, Wilber R, Zink RC, Cross A, Colonno A, Fernandes L. 2006. Entecavir versus lamivudine for patients with chronic hepatitis B. *New England Journal of Medicine*, 354(10), 1011-1020.

[39] Leung N, Peng CY, Hann HW, Sollano J, Lao-Tan J, Hsu CW, Lesmana L, Yuen MF, Jeffers L, Sherman M, Min A, Mencarini K, Diva U, Cross A, Wilber R, Lopez-Talavera J. 2009. Early hepatitis B virus DNA reduction in hepatitis B e antigen-positive patients with chronic hepatitis B: A randomized international study of entecavir versus adefovir. *Hepatology*, 49(1), 72-79.

[40] Chang TT, Liaw YF, Wu SS, Schiff E, Han KH, Lai CL, Safadi R, Lee SS, Halota W, Goodman Z, Chi YC, Zhang H, Hindes R, Iloeje U, Beebe S, Kreter B. 2010. Long-term entecavir therapy results in the reversal of fibrosis/cirrhosis and continued histological improvement in patients with chronic hepatitis B. *Hepatology*, 52(3), 886-893.

[41] Tenney DJ, Rose RE, Baldick CK, Pokornowski KA, Eggers BJ, Fang J, Wichroski MJ, Xu D, Yang J, Wilber RB, Colonno RJ. 2009. Long-term monitoring shows hepatitis B virus resistance to entecavir in nucleoside-naïve patients is rare through five years of therapy. *Hepatology*, 49(5), 1503-1515.

[42] Locarnini S. 2008. Primary resistance, multidrug resistance, and cross-resistance pathways in HBV as a consequence of treatment failure. *Hepatology International*, 2(2), 147-151.

[43] Lai CL, Gane E, Liaw YF, Hsu CW, Thongsawat S, Wang Y, Chen Y, Heathcote EJ, Rasenack J, Bsowej N, Naoumov NV, DiBisceglie AM, Zeuzem S, Moon YM, Goodman Z, Chao G, Constance BF, Brown NA. 2007. Telbivudine versus lamivudine in patients with chronic hepatitis B. *New England Journal of Medicine*, 357(25), 2576-2588.

[44] Liaw YF, Gane E, Leung N, Zeuzem S, Wang Y, Lai CL, Heathcote EJ, Manns M, Bzowej N, Niu J, Han SH, Hwang SG, Cakaloglu Y, Tong MJ Papatheodoridis G, Chen Y, Brown NA, Albanis E, Galil K, Naoumov NV. 2-year GLOBE trial results: telbuvidine is superior to lamivudine in patients with chronic hepatitis B. *Gastroenterology*, 136(2), 486-495.

[45] Gane EJ, Wang Y, Liaw YF, Hou J, Thongsawat S, Wan M, Moon YM, Jia J, Chao YC, Niu J, Leung N, Samuel D, Hsu CW, Bao W, Lopez P, Avila C. 2011. Efficacy and safety of prolonged 3-year telbuvidine treatment in patients with chronic hepatitis B. *Liver International*, 31(5), 676-684.

[46] Chan HL, Heathcote EJ, Marcellin P, Lai CL, Cho M, Moon YM, Chao YC, Myers RP, Minuk GY, Jeffers L, Sievert W, Bzowej N, Harb G, Kaiser R, Qiao XJ, Brown NA. 2007. Treatment of hepatitis e antigen chronic hepatitis with telbivudine or adefovir: A randomized trial. *Annals of Internal Medicine*, 147(11), 745-754.

[47] Fung J, Lai C-L, Seto W-K, Yuen M-F. 2011. Nucleoside/nucleotide analogues in the treatment of chronic hepatitis B. *Journal of Antimicrobial Chemotherapy*, 66)12, 2715-2725.

[48] Marcellin P, Heathcote EK, Buti M, Gane E, de Man RA, Krastev Z, Germanidis G, Lee SS, Flisiak R, Kaita K, Manns M, Kotzev I, Tchernev K, Buggisch P, Weilert F, Kurdas OO, Shiffman ML, Trinh H, Washington MK, Sorbel J, Anderson J, Snow-Lampart A, Mondou E, Quinn J, Rousseau F. 2008. Tenofovir disoproxil fumarate versus adefovir dipivoxil for chronic hepatitis B. *New England Journal of Medicine*, 359(23), 2442-2455.

[49] Marcellin P, Buti M, Gane EJ, Krastev Z, Flisiak R, Germanidis G, Washington MK, Barnes CN, Flaherty JF, Bornstein JD, McHutchinson JG, Heathcote EJ. 2011. Five years of treatment with tenofovir DF (TDF) for chronic hepatitis B (CHB) infection is associated with sustained viral suppression and significant regression of histological fibrosis and cirrhosis. 62nd Annual Meeting of the American Association for the Study of Liver Disease (AASLD 2011). San Francisco, November 4-8, 2011. Abstract 1375.

[50] Lam Y-F, Yuen M-F, Seto W-K, Lai C-L. 2011. Current antiviral therapy of chronic hepatitis B: efficacy and safety. *Current Hepatitis Reports*, 10(4), 235-243.

[51] Segovia MC, Chacra W, Gordon SC. 2012. Adefovir dipivoxil in chronic hepatitis B: history and current uses. *Expert Opinion on Pharmacotherapy*, 13(2), 245-254.

[52] Fernandez-Fernandez B, Montoya-Ferrer A, Sanz AB, Sanchez-Nino MD, Izquierdo MC, Poveda J, Sainz-Prestel V, Ortiz-Martin N, Parra-Rodriguez A, Selgas R, Ruiz-Ortega M, Egido J, Ortiz A. 2011. Tenofovir nephrotoxicity: 2011 update. *AIDS Research and Treatment*. Epub 2011 June 7.

[53] Lange CM, Bojunga J, Hofmann WP, Wunder K, Mihm U, Zeuzem S, Sarrazin C. 2009. Severe lactic acidosis during treatment of chronic hepatitis B with entecavir in patients with impaired liver function. *Hepatology*, 50(6), 2001-2006.

[54] Zoulim F, Locarnini S. 2012. Management of treatment failure in chronic hepatitis B. *Journal of Hepatology*, 56(1), S112-122.

[55] Gish R, Jia JD, Locarnini S, Zoulim F. 2012. Selection of chronic hepatitis B therapy with high barrier to resistance. *Lancet Infectious Diseases*.

[56] Massoumi H, Martin P, Tan H-H. 2011. Management of chronic hepatitis B. *European Journal of Gastroenterology and Hepatology*, 23(8), 642-650.

[57] Keeffe EB, Dieterich DT, Han SH, Jacobson IM, Martin P, Schiff ER, Tobias H. 2008. A treatment algorithm for the management of hepatitis B virus infection in the United States: 2008 update. *Clinical Gastroenterology and Hepatology*, 6(12), 1315-1341.

[58] Lok AS, McMahon BJ. 2009. Chronic hepatitis B: Update 2009, *Hepatology*, 50(3), 1-36.

[59] Marcellin P, Dusheiko G, Zoulim F, Esteban R, Hadziyannis S, Lamertico P, Manns M, Shouval D, Yurdaydin C. 2009. EASL clinical practice guidelines: Management of chronic hepatitis B. *Journal of Hepatology*, 50, 222-242.

[60] Liaw YF, Leung N, Kao JH, Piratvisuth T, Gane E, Han KH, Guan R, Lau GK, Locarnini S. 2008. Asian-Pacific consensus statement on the management of chronic hepatitis B: a 2008 update. *Hepatology International*, 2(3), 263-283.

In: Hepatitis B: New Research
Editors: J. T. Cox and D. I. Owen
ISBN 978-1-62081-846-6

Chapter V

Hepatitis B Virus Infection among Middle School Students in South Brazil: Epidemiology and Vaccination

Ana Maria Passos[1], Aricio Treitinger[2] and Celso Spada[2]
[1]Clinical Virology Laboratory, Division of Infectious Diseases, Federal University of Sao Paulo, Brazil
[2]Department of Clinical Analysis, Health Sciences Center, Federal University of Santa Catarina, Brazil

Abstract

Introduction. Hepatitis B virus (HBV) infection is still a major public health problem in Brazil. It is estimated that at least 15% of the population has been exposed to HBV. Hepatitis B is unequally distributed throughout the country, as a result of the wide territory and socio-economic differences. Hepatitis B vaccination in South Brazil began in 1993, limited to children younger than 4 years of age. Currently, it is recommended in a three-dose schedule beginning at birth. Vaccination against HBV is also available for unvaccinated persons up to 29 years. Objectives. The aim of this study was to determine the prevalence of hepatitis B markers of infection and immunity among middle school students in the state of Santa Catarina, Brazil. *Patients and methods.* This comprehensive cross-sectional seroprevalence study included 2,044 volunteers aged 10 to 16 years old in five major cities of the state. From 2008 to 2009 blood samples were obtained from all enrolled subjects and stored at –20ºC. HBsAg, anti-HBc and anti-HBs serologies were performed using automated microparticles enzymatic immunoassay (Abbott®, AxSYM System). Previously published results will be analyzed along with new data. *Results.* The overall prevalence of present or past HBV infection in the studied population was 0.9% (18 subjects). Eighty eight percent (88%) of all adolescents had detectable anti-HBs titers and 11% presented susceptibility to HBV infection, with no seromarkers for HBV. *Conclusion.* This study found a very low prevalence of HBV markers of infection and a great percentage of immunity, demonstrating the success of the vaccination program against hepatitis B in the state. These findings preindicate a very optimistic situation as to HBV infection and its consequences in the future for this population. With this continuous decrease in rates of HBV, public health resources could be redirected from treating HBV-related conditions to treating other diseases that cannot be so easily prevented.

Introduction

Hepatitis B virus (HBV) infection is a problem of global health importance and represents a significant cause of morbidity and mortality worldwide. HBV can be transmitted parenterally, sexually and perinatally. Despite progress on prophylaxis, diagnostic and treatment of HBV infection, it remains one of the major causes of chronic liver disease, cirrhosis or hepatocellular carcinoma [1].

The World Health Organization estimates that more than two billion of the global population has been infected with HBV, and out of these, approximately 360 million are chronically infected and at risk for HBV-related liver disease. Approximately one third of all cases of cirrhosis and half of all cases of hepatocellular carcinoma can be attributed to chronic HBV infection. HBV is estimated to be responsible for 500,000 to 700,000 deaths each year worldwide [2].

The prevalence of HBV carriers varies from 0.1 percent to 2 percent in low prevalence areas (United States and Canada, Western Europe, Australia and New Zealand), to 3 to 5 percent in intermediate prevalence areas (Mediterranean countries, Japan, Central Asia, Middle East, and Latin and

South America), to 10 to 20 percent in high prevalence areas (southeast Asia, China, sub-Saharan Africa) [3].

The wide range in HBV carrier rates in different parts of the world is largely related to differences in the age at infection, which is inversely related to the risk of chronicity. The rate of progression from acute to chronic HBV infection is approximately 90 percent for perinatally acquired infection, 20 to 50 percent for infections between the age of 1 and 5 years and less than 5 percent for adult acquired infection [4].

HBV infection is still a public health problem in Brazil and estimates indicate that at least 15% of the population has been exposed to HBV [1]. Hepatitis B is unequally distributed throughout the country, as a result of the wide territory and socioeconomic differences. Certain areas have a higher HBV prevalence, such as the western Amazon and even some parts of southern Brazil.

Hepatitis B infection and chronic carriage acquisition is preventable with safe and effective vaccines that have been available since 1982 and are now the most widely used vaccines in the world. They contain a non-infectious viral particle that contains purified surface antigen (HBsAg) of the virus. Early vaccines were plasma-derived. Second generation vaccines are produced by recombinant DNA technology using modified yeast cultures. The vaccine is given as a series of three intramuscular doses. Studies have shown that three doses of HepB vaccine are 95% effective in preventing children and adults from developing chronic infection if they have not yet been infected. Efficacy is long lasting [3].

Hepatitis B vaccination began in 1989 in some regions of Brazil, directed primarily to specific groups. Some years later (1998), it became available in more regions and to children aged below one year old, as well as to high-risk population. Afterwards, the coverage of the vaccine was extended to health students, military and adolescents up to 15 years old. In South Brazil, hepatitis B vaccination began in 1993, limited to children younger than 4 years of age [5]. Currently, it is recommended in a three-dose schedule beginning at birth. Vaccination against HBV is also available for unvaccinated persons up to 29 years.

It is well known that during the ages between 10 and 16, there is an increase of risk practices that can lead to HBV infection, such as unprotected sexual relations, tattooing and body piercing. Knowing the actual prevalence of HBV infection and immunity in adolescents is important for the evaluation and improvement of current prevention strategies. The aim of this study was to determine the prevalence of hepatitis B markers of infection and immunity among middle school students in the state of Santa Catarina, Brazil.

Patients and Methods

This comprehensive cross-sectional seroprevalence study was undertaken to determine the prevalence of HBV markers and vaccine coverage in adolescents in Santa Catarina. The studied population consisted of middle school students aged 10 to 16 years old, attending public or private schools.

Five major cities in the state were selected for the study: Florianópolis (state capital), Chapecó, Lages, Blumenau and Itajaí. They are located in the east coast, west region, mountain region and in the valley, respectively.

To successfully estimate the prevalence of HBV infection markers in this population a minimum sample of 322 volunteers in each city was calculated to be sufficient at a 95% confidence interval (CI) and 0.05 alpha error (using an expected probability of prevalence of approximately 30%).

A random sampling plan was conducted for the selection of volunteers so that it would reproduce the distribution of the adolescent population in middle school in each city of the study, including the administrative category of school attendance (public or private), their dimension and geographic locations in the city.

Approval for the study was obtained from the Ethics Committee of the Federal University of Santa Catarina (protocols 351/06, 238/07, 284/07, 260/07, 171/09) and written informed consent was obtained from a parent or legal guardian of all participants.

Vaccination cards were checked in order to assess coverage characteristics including vaccination status and number of doses received.

From 2008 to 2009, blood samples were obtained from all enrolled subjects and stored at –20ºC. HBsAg, anti-HBc and anti-HBs serologies were obtained, and each test was performed using automated microparticles enzymatic immunoassay (Abbott®, AxSYM System). HbsAg and anti-HBc results were categorized as either "positive" or "negative" according to the provided cut-offs. Anti-HBs titers were categorized as "undetectable" if anti-HBs was less than the cut-off value, "detectable" if anti-HBs was less than 10IU/L, and "reactive" if anti-HBs was greater than or equal to 10IU/L, according to the manufacturer's instructions.

Statistics included Pearson's chi-square test for the comparison of categorical values using a significance lever of $p<0.050$. All data were entered into and analyzed using SPSS version 11.0 (SPSS Inc., Chicago, IL, USA).

Published results from Florianópolis [6], Chapecó [7], Itajaí [8] and Blumenau [9, 10] will be analyzed collectively, from now on, along with new unpublished data.

Results

A total of 2,044 adolescents were enrolled in this study.

The overall prevalence of present or past HBV infection in the studied population was 0.9% (18 subjects) and did not differ statistically between males (1.3%) and females (0.6%), or among the 5 cities surveyed (Florianópolis 0.5%, Blumenau 1%, Itajaí 1%, Chapecó 1%, Lages 0.9%).

Eighty eight percent (88%) of all adolescents had detectable anti-HBs titers and 11% presented susceptibility to HBV infection, with no seromarkers for HBV. Detailed information on the prevalence of HBV markers in the studied population is presented in Table 1.

Vaccination coverage was 99% and 94% of all subjects completed the 3-dose schedule. In all, 88% presented anti-HBs antibodies. Fifty-four per cent (54%) had reactive anti-HBs titers, 34% had detectable antibodies, and 12% had undetectable anti-HBs. When considering only those who completed the 3-dose vaccination schedule, percentages for anti-HBs titers were 56%, 34% and 10%, respectively.

Table 1. Seroprevalence of HBV markers in middle school students in South Brazil

HBV markers	Number	Percentage
HBsAg (+), anti-HBc (–), anti-HBs (–)	1	0.05
HBsAg (–), anti-HBc (+), anti-HBs (–)	1	0.05
HBsAg (+), anti-HBc (+), anti-HBs (–)	5	0.3
HBsAg (–), anti-HBc (+), anti-HBs (+)	11	0.5
HBsAg (–), anti-HBc (–), anti-HBs (+)	1793	87.7
HBsAg (–), anti-HBc (–), anti-HBs (–)	233	11.4

Discussion

A very low prevalence of present or past HBV infection was found among the middle school students in South Brazil.

Other prevalence studies in Brazil have found low prevalence of HBV infection markers. Miranda *et al.* established the prevalence of hepatitis B serological markers among 632 individuals submitted to blood tests in health centers of Ribeirao Preto, Sao Paulo. They found an HbsAg prevalence of 0.3% and an anti-HBc prevalence of 13.9%. However, there was no case of positive anti-HBc in the age group of 10 to 19 years old [11].

Furthermore, the prevalence of HBV infection markers has decreased in the last years. Silveira *et al.* conducted a study of hepatitis B seroprevalence in Latin America from 1994 to 1997. They described a wide range of HBV seroprevalence in different regions of Brazil, with a high rate in Manaus (21%), followed by Porto Alegre (7.5%), Rio de Janeiro (5.5%), and Fortaleza (1.2%) [12]. Rosini *et al.* estimated the prevalence of serological markers for HBV infection among blood donors in Santa Catarina in the years of 1999, 2000 and 2001. They found HBsAg prevalence of 0.98% (1999), 0.84% (2000) and 0.64% (2001), and anti-HBc prevalence of 8.83% (1999), 7.09% (2000) and 5.35% (2001) [13].

Recently, the Brazilian Ministry of Health, with aid of some Federal Universities, conducted a seroprevalence study about viral hepatitis in state capitals nationwide. Results from Northeast, Central region and Federal District, from 2004 to 2005, among 13 to 19 years old non-vaccinated individuals (3.5%, 2.2% and 1.6%, respectively) and among vaccinated individuals (1.3%, 1.5% and 1.3%, respectively) have been presented [14].

The prevalence of HBV infection found in this study is similar to the one reported in Portugal for adolescents with a mean age of 14 years old (0.6%) and that reported in Italy for individuals up to 24 years old (1.0%); but it is inferior to the one reported in first time eligible blood-donors from North, Northeast and Southeast Brazil (2.9%) and to the one found in blood donors in South Brazil (15,6%) [15-18].

This low prevalence of HBV markers of infection found in this study may be a reflection of low HBV circulation among subjects in this age group probably due to the recent efforts in vaccinating infants and adolescents up to 24 years old in Brazil, which can be reinforced by the anti-HBs prevalence here found.

The results found in our study are in part justified by these facts, since a significant proportion (54%) of volunteers presented anti-HBs titers greater than or equal to 10IU/L and were, therefore, considered immunized against hepatitis B. Of the excessively, 34% presented detectable titers below 10IU/L and 12% presented undetectable titers of anti-HBs. The overall prevalence of anti-HBs antibodies was 88%; vaccination coverage was 99%, and 94% of all subjects completed the 3-dose schedule.

Since the hepatitis B vaccine was included in the Brazilian National Immunization Program, there has been a substantial increase in vaccination coverage, especially among children and adolescents. Mandatory screening has reduced the transmission of HBV through blood transfusions, but sexual transmission remains a concern among unvaccinated adolescents and adults. This raises questions regarding the need to promote vaccination through educational campaigns, whether the vaccination strategy has been adequate, and whether vaccination coverage is high enough to decrease the occurrence of disease [19, 20].

The coverage rate found in this study almost reaches that expected by the Brazilian Ministry of Health (95%), demonstrating the efficacy of current vaccination policies for children.

Several studies argue about the necessity of booster doses of the vaccine for those with anti- HBs detectable titers below 10 UI/L. Also, there are authors who suggest that strong immunologic memory persists for more than 10 years once the complete vaccination scheme has been administered properly and therefore, an anamnestic anti-HBs response is achieved after HBV contact, even if anti-HBs titers are not higher than 10IU/L [21-23]. Thus, considering that the great majority of the adolescents studied have been vaccinated over 10 years ago, and that 94% completed the HepB 3-dose schedule, one may consider that real immunity ranges from 88% to 94% (prevalence of anti-HBs antibodies and 3-dose HepB vaccine coverage, respectively).

As expected, the anti-HBs prevalence found in this study is higher than that of 57% found by our group among young adults (ranging from 18 to 19 years old) born prior to the full implementation of the HBV vaccination program [24]. Additionally, it was similar to that of Italy, in which among 1,212 vaccinated children (mean age 10.9 years), 91% presented detectable anti-HBs antibodies [22].

Although the reality described here cannot be extrapolated to older age groups in the region studied, the observations made reveal that a successful vaccination strategy will result in a population of adults protected against

HBV, within a few years, with prevalence rates in this age group that are also similar to that of developed countries. This high vaccine coverage will also have an impact on lowering future hepatic cancer rates in this population, thus allowing public health economic resources to be spent in less preventable illnesses.

Conclusion

This study found a very low prevalence of HBV markers of infection and a great percentage of immunity, demonstrating the success of the vaccination program against hepatitis B in the state. These findings preindicate a very optimistic situation as to HBV infection and its consequences in the future for this population. With this continuous decrease in rates of HBV, public health resources could be redirected from treating HBV-related conditions to treating other diseases that cannot be so easily prevented.

References

[1] World Health Organization. Global distribution of hepatitis A, B and C, 2001. *Weekly Epidemiological Record*, 2002, v. 77, n. 6, p. 46-47.

[2] World Health Organization. Hepatitis B vaccines. *Weekly Epidemiological Record*, 2009, v. 84, n. 40, p. 405-420.

[3] Shepard, CW; Simard, EP; Finelli, L; Fiore, AE; Bell, BP. Hepatitis B virus infection: epidemiology and vaccination. *Epidemiologic Reviews*, 2006, v. 28, n. 1, p. 112-125.

[4] McMahon, BJ. Natural history of chronic hepatitis B - clinical implications. *The Medscape Journal of Medicine*, 2008, v. 10, n. 4, p. 91.

[5] Brazilian Ministry of Health. National immunization program: 30 years. Brasilia, Brazil: Ministry of Health; 2003.

[6] Voigt, AR; Strazer Neto, M; Spada, C; Treitinger, A. Seroprevalence of hepatitis B and hepatitis C markers among children and adolescents in the south Brazilian region—metropolitan area of Florianopolis, Santa Catarina. *Brazilian Journal of Infectious Diseases*, 2010, v. 14, n. 1, p. 60-65.

[7] Scaraveli, NG; Passos, AM; Voigt, AR; Livramento, A; Tonial, G; Treitinger, A; Spada, C. Seroprevalence of hepatitis B and hepatitis C markers in adolescents in South- ern Brazil. Cadernos de Saude Publica, 2011, v. 27, n. 4, p. 753-758.

[8] Tonial, GC; Passos, AM; Livramento, A; Scaraveli, NG; Batschauer, APB; Bueno, EC; Largura, A; Spada, C; Treitinger, A. Hepatitis B markers seroprevalence and vaccination coverage in adoles- cents in Southern Brazil. Revista da Sociedade Brasileira de Medicina Tropical, 2011, v. 44, n. 4, p. 416-419.

[9] Livramento, A; Córdova, CMM; Spada, C; Treitinger, A. Seroprevalence of hepatitis B and C infection markers among children and adolescents in the southern Brazilian region. Revista do Instituto de Medicina Tropical de Sao Paulo, 2011, v. 53, n. 1, p. 13-17.

[10] Livramento, A; Córdova, CMM; Scaraveli, NG; Tonial, GC; Spada, C; Treitinger, A. Anti-HBs levels among children and adolescents with complete immunization schedule against hepatitis B virus. A cross-sectional study in Blumenau, State of Santa Catarina, Brazil, 2007-2008. Revista da Sociedade Brasileira de Medicina Tropical, v. 44, n. 4, p. 412-415.

[11] Miranda, LVG; Passos, ADC; Figueiredo, JFC; Gaspar, AMC; Yoshida, CFT. [Serological markers of hepatitis B in people submitted to blood testing in health care clinics]. Revista de Saude Publica, 2000, v. 34, n. 3, p. 286-291.

[12] Silveira, TR; Fonseca, JC; Rivera, L; Fay, OH; Tapia, R; Santos, JI; Urdeneta, E; Clemens, SAC. Hepatitis B seroprevalence in Latin America. *Pan American Journal of Publich Health*, 1999, v. 6, n. 6, p. 378-383.

[13] Rosini, N; Mousse, D; Spada, C; Treitinger, A. Seroprevalence of HBsAg, anti-HBc and anti-HCV in Southern Brazil, 1999- 2001. *Brazilian Journal of Infectious Diseases*, 2003, v. 7, n. 4, p. 262-267.

[14] Pereira, LM; Martelli, CM; Merchán-Hamann, E; Montarroyos, UR; Braga, MC; de Lima, ML; Cardoso, MR; Turchi, MD; Costa, MA; de Alencar, LC; Moreira, RC; Figueiredo, GM; Ximenes, RA; Hepatitis Study Group. Population-based multicentric survey of hepatitis B infection and risk factor differences among three regions in Brazil. *American Journal of Tropical and Medical Hygiene*, 2009, v. 81, n. 2, p. 240-247.

[15] Antunes, H; Macedo, M; Estrada, A. [Hepatitis B virus vaccination rate with immunization]. Acta Medica Portuguesa, 2004, v. 17, n. 4, p. 303-308.

[16] Fabris, P; Baldo, V; Baldovin, T; Bellotto, E; Rassu, M; Trivello, R; Tramarin, A; Tositti, G; Floreani, A. Changing epidemiology of HCV and HBV infections in Northern Italy: a survey in the general population. *Journal of Clinical Gastroenterology*, 2008, v. 42, n. 5, p. 527-32.

[17] Nascimento, MC; Mayaud, P; Sabino, EC; Torres, KL; Franceschi, S. Prevalence of hepatitis B and C serological markers among first-time blood donors in Brazil: a multi-center serosurvey. *Journal of Medical Virology*, 2008, v. 80, n. 1, p.53-57.

[18] Martelli, CM; Turchi, M; Souto, FJ; Sáez-Alquézar, A; Andrade, AL; Zicker, F. Anti-HBc testing for blood donations in areas with intermediate hepatitis B endemicity. *Pan American Journal of Public Health*, 1999, v. 6, n. 1, p. 69-73.

[19] Luna, EJ; Veras, MA; Flannery, B; de Moraes, JC. Household survey of hepatitis B vaccine coverage among Brazilian children. *Vaccine*, 2009, v. 27, n. 39, p. 5326-5331.

[20] National Sanitary Regulatory Agency (ANVISA). Report on the National Blood Surveillance System . Brasília, Brazil: Ministry of Health; 2009.

[21] Banatvala, JE; Van Damme, P. Hepatitis B vaccine – do we need boosters? *Journal of Viral Hepatology*, 2003, v. 10, n. 1, p. 1-6.

[22] Zanetti, AR; Mariano, A; Romanò, L; D'Amelio, R; Chironna, M; Coppola, RC; Cuccia, M; Mangione, R; Marrone, F; Negrone, FS; Parlato, A; Zamparo, E; Zotti, C; Stroffolini, T; Mele, A; Study Group. Long-term immunogenicity of hepatitis B vaccination and policy for booster: an Italian multicentre study. *Lancet*, 2005, v. 366, n. 9494, p. 1379-1384.

[23] But DY, Lai CL, Lim WL, Fung J, Wong DK, Yuen MF. Twenty-two years follow-up of a prospective randomized trial of hepatitis B vaccines without booster dose in children: final report. *Vaccine*, 2008, v. 26, n. 51, p. 6587-6591.

[24] Passos, AM; Treitinger, A; Spada, C. Hepatitis B immunity and vaccination coverage among young adult males in the Air Force in South Brazil. *Vaccine*, 2011, v. 29, n. 49, p. 9284-9288.

In: Hepatitis B: New Research
Editors: J. T. Cox and D. I. Owen
ISBN 978-1-62081-846-6

Chapter VI

Challenges in Risk Assessment for Hepatocellular Carcinoma: Example of Hepatitis B Virus Infection

***Myriam Lereau*[1,2]*, Doriane Gouas*[2]*, Nora Martel*[1]*, Tatiana Dupinay*[1] *and Isabelle Chemin*[1]**
[1]Université Lyon 1, France,
Centre de Recherche en Cancérologie de Lyon, Lyon, France
[2]International Agency for Research on Cancer, Lyon, France

Abstract

A number of risk factors appear to play a role in hepatocellular carcinoma (HCC), hepatitis B infection being one of the most important. Hepatitis B surface antigen (HBsAg) is the hallmark of hepatitis B virus (HBV) since it is the best and most reliable diagnostic marker. However, since most studies do not rely on longitudinal observations but mostly on cross-sectional studies little is known on time changes in those markers and their incidence. Chronic inflammation and cytokines are key determinants in the development of fibrosis and liver cell proliferation. Integration of HBV DNA into host cellular DNA is crucial during HBV chronic infection by disrupting or promoting expression of cellular genes that are important in cell growth and differentiation. In addition, expression of HBV proteins may have a direct effect on cellular functions, and some of these gene products can promote malignant transformation. Several HBV genes have been found in infected tumoral tissues more frequently than others, including truncated pre-S2/S and hepatitis B X genes. The proteins expressed from these integrated genes have been shown to have intracellular activities that may account for their association with HCC, including effects on cellular growth and apoptosis. A major player involved in this form of viral transactivation is the X protein (HBx) that displays pleiotropic functions and has been implicated in the malignant transformation of chronically-infected liver cells. Occult hepatitis B virus infection is characterized by persistence of HBV DNA in HBsAg-negative individuals. There are evidences that occult HBV constitutes a risk factor for the development of HCC and that the mechanisms whereby overt HBV might induce tumor formation are maintained in those atypical HBV infections.

Introduction

Chronic hepatitis B virus (HBV) infection is a primary risk factor for the development of cirrhosis and hepatocellular carcinoma (HCC) worldwide. HBV carriers are identified by detection of the hepatitis B virus surface antigen (HBsAg) in their blood and persistence of HBsAg over a time interval of 6 months defines chronic hepatitis B.

If HBsAg detection means ongoing HBV infection its disappearance may have different meanings either true clearance of the virus or just its decline to low grade persisting occult HBV infection. Moreover, co-infection of HBV with HIV or HCV could lead to down-regulation of HBsAg production or interference with its detection.

It has indeed become evident through a large number of studies that HBV may persist in the form of serologically silent infections, leading to the concept of seronegative or occult infection. In a recent expert guideline, occult HBV infection (OBI) has been defined as the presence of HBV DNA in the liver, in the absence of HBsAg and with low titers or even absence of HBV DNA in serum. Such infection may significantly contribute to the population burden of HBV-related diseases since occult HBV infections are spread worldwide. Many studies have been carried out on OBI in different parts of the world since the early 1980s. Some of these studies have suggested that OBI may play a role in chronic liver damage and in the development of HCC, particularly in patients with chronic hepatitis C.

It is to note that both integrated viral DNA and covalently closed circular HBV genomes (HBV cccDNA) are present in the liver of patients with OBI, and the persistence of free viral genomes is associated with continuance of viral transcription and replication. Thus, the direct and indirect mechanisms whereby overt HBV may induce tumor formation appear to be mostly maintained by OBI.

HBV Presentation

Structure of the Genome

Human hepatitis B virus (HBV) is a small enveloped DNA virus belonging to the *Hepadnavidiae* family. One unique feature is that the viral genome is a non-covalently closed circular DNA of about 3.2kb with a partially double-stranded region over 50% to 80% of its length, giving rise to a relaxed circular DNA (RC DNA) (Figure 1A).

The (-) strand is complete and contains the entire genetic inheritance of the virus; a viral polymerase is covalently linked to its 5' end. The (+) strand is incomplete, with a fixed 5' end and a variable 3' end; it overlaps the 5' and 3' of the (-) strand, thus ensuring the genomic circularity.

Four overlapping open reading frames (ORF) encode the 7 viral proteins:

- The C gene encodes the pre-core protein or HBe antigen (HBeAg) and the capsid/core protein or HBcAg;
- The S gene encodes the 3 surface proteins: L (large), M (medium) and S (small, HBsAg);
- The P gene encodes the viral polymerase;
- And the X gene is the smallest ORF and encodes HBxAg.

Besides the splicing events of mRNAs, HBV increases its genetic complexity by using different initiation sites of transcription. Moreover, alternative codons for initiation of the protein synthesis allow generating several proteins from one single ORF, as for HBeAg/HBcAg and the three surface proteins.

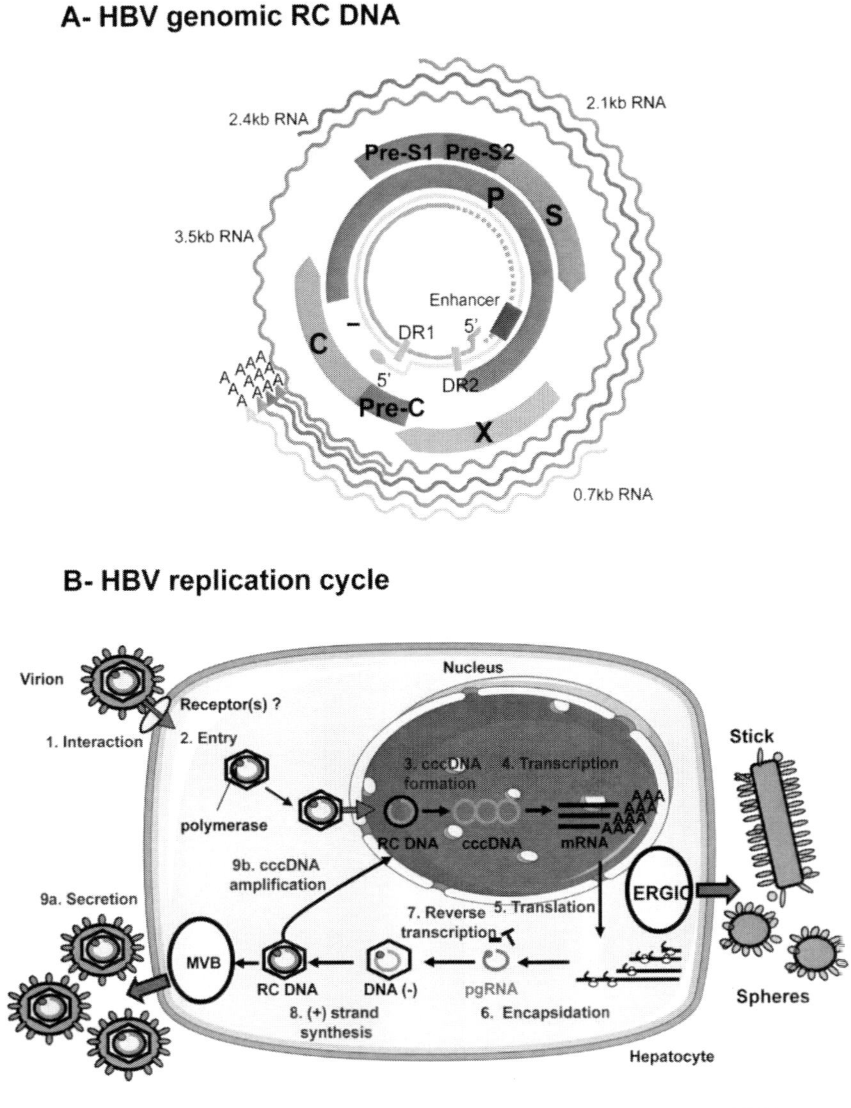

Figure 1. HBV characteristics. (A) Structure of HBV genomic DNA. HBV genome contains the four ORF S, P, C and X. The corresponding mRNAs and lengths are indicated in the same colors as genes. Adapted from Jay H. Hoofnagle, 2002. (B) HBV replication cycle. Nine steps describe the life cycle of the virus, which ends in secretion of infectious particles through MVB or secretion of non-infectious particles (spheres and sticks) through ERGIC. MVB: Multi-Vesicular Bodies; ERGIC: Endoplasmic Reticulum-Golgi Intermediate Compartment. The cell was drawn thanks to Servier Medical Art (http://www.servier.fr/smart/home_smart.asp).

Replication Cycle

HBV is also qualified as a DNA para-retrovirus as its replication cycle contains a retro-transcription step.

The cycle starts with the entry of the infectious particle, also called virion, into the hepatocyte by endocytose (Figure 1B). The mechanism of entry has not been completely elucidated so far. However several studies suggest that it would be mediated by interactions between viral envelope proteins and two types of cellular receptors at the surface [1]: the first type would be of high affinity and the second type of low affinity would belong to heparan sulfate proteoglycans. Moreover Leistner et al. proposed a model: *in vivo* HBV would be initially trapped in the liver in the space of Dissé by heparan sulfate proteoglycans, then bind to a high affinity receptor through the pre-S1 attachment site and the N-terminal myristic acid [2]. After the fusion of the viral envelop with the cell membrane, the nucleocapsid is released into the cytoplasm. Then a model has been set up from *in vitro* studies: the capsid would be directed *via* the microtubules to the center of microtubule organization which is located in the periphery of the nucleus; the capsid contains a NLS sequence which would allow its interaction with importin α and β and facilitate its translocation into the nuclear pore; finally the capsid would be dismantled into HBcAg dimers inside the pore, allowing the release of the genomic RC DNA into the nucleus [3]. Once inside the nucleus, the RC DNA undergoes several modifications before being converted into a very stable double-stranded covalently-closed circular DNA (cccDNA). This cccDNA forms a "mini-chromosome" which serves as a viral "tank" inside the infected cells: it is transcribed by the cellular RNA polymerase into different mRNAs and pre-genomic RNA (pgRNA), the latter being the mRNA of the entire genome. mRNAs are translated in the endoplasmic reticulum into different viral proteins which are able to assemble into new viral particles. The pgRNA is then encapsided with the viral polymerase and cellular heat shock proteins [4]. Inside the capsid the polymerase has several enzymatic activities to convert the pgRNA into RC DNA: it serves as primer for the (-) strand synthesis, retro-transcriptase, RNase H and DNA-dependent DNA polymerase [5]. Finally the nucleocapsid containing the neo-synthesized RC DNA can be directed either to multi-vesicular bodies to be matured and secreted after association with envelop proteins and insertion into the cell membrane in order to form new infection particles [6], or to the nucleus in order to amplify the cccDNA pool. In parallel, the viral DNA can also integrate into the host genome in a relatively random way as fragments of variable length.

Viral Proteins: Role in HCC

Hepatocarcinogenesis mediated by HBV is associated with the chronicity of infection. The evolution of HBV infection towards chronicity depends on the age and the immune system of the individual at the time of infection: 5 to 10% of immune-competent individuals and 90% of newborns or children develop a chronic infection [7]. The mechanisms responsible for the malignant transformation during a chronic infection by HBV involve host and viral factors. HBV is not cytophatic by itself but liver injuries caused by chronic HBV infection are considered to be immune-mediated. Moreover a direct role of the virus in hepatocarcinogenesis is well established. However, it is not known whether the viral infection causes the initiation of the tumor or the subsequent inflammation leading to liver regenèration and to cirrhosis acts as a tumorous promoter in hepatocarcinogenesis. Several studies suggest that some viral proteins, especially surface proteins and HBxAg, may contribute to HBV-induced carcinogenesis by interacting with host factors leading to an alteration of cellular gene expression. Nevertheless, the role of these proteins through direct or indirect mechanisms is still not clear.

Surface Proteins: Endoplasmic Reticulum Stress

Expression of the various types of surface proteins depends on the replicative status of the HBV genome. During the acute phase of HBV infection, HBsAg is predominant. On the contrary, during the chronic phase, the HBV genome integrates into the host genome and the L protein becomes predominant. A number of truncated surface genes with a partially deleted pre-S1 or pre-S2 region have already been identified and may contribute to HCC development by accumulating in the endoplasmic reticulum (ER) and inducing ER stress [8]. ΔS-L mutants from L protein are frequently detected in the serum of chronically infected patients [9]. Studies have shown that the weaker the viral replication is, the more these mutants appear and this evolution could be a consequence of the host immune pressure [10]. Moreover, ΔS-L mutants have been shown to accumulate in the ER and induce genomic instability by generating an oxidative stress, DNA damage and mutations [8].

HBx Protein: The Super-HBV Gangster in HCC

HBx is a regulatory protein of 154 amino acids known to exhibit a transcriptional transactivation function. Previous observations suggest that HBx has two independent cell proliferative (pro-oncogenic domain) and death-promoting (pro-apoptotic domain) activities (Figure 2). Since HBx has no

DNA-binding activity, it exerts these functions through interaction with cellular factor(s). Nevertheless, how HBx operates in cellular transformation remains unclear.

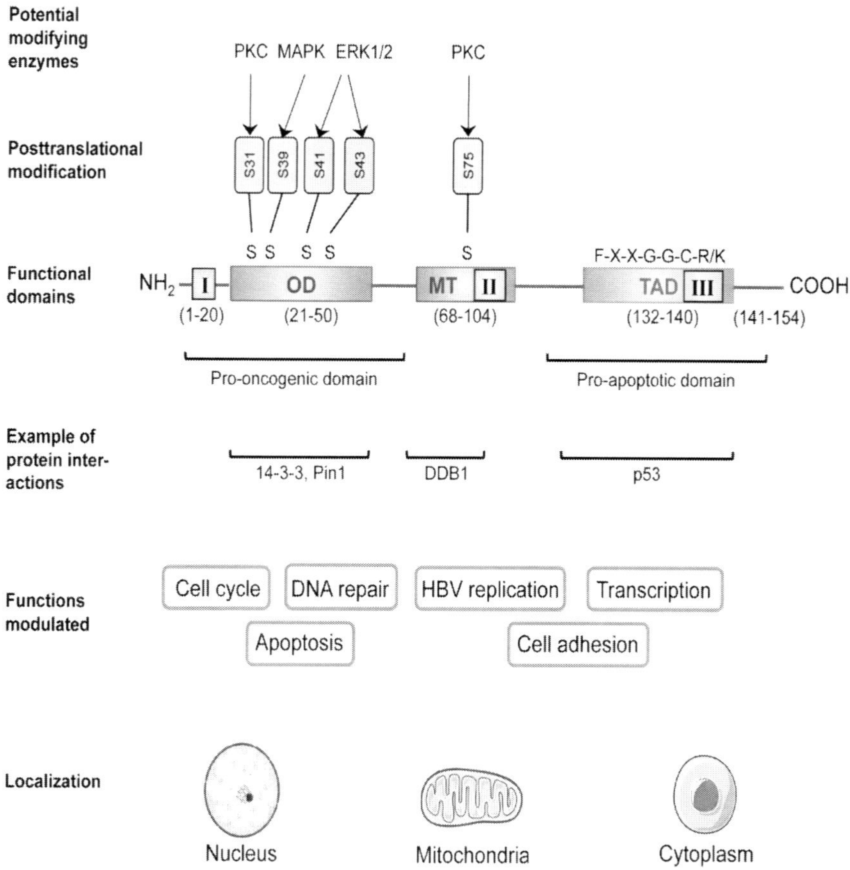

Figure 2. Structure, posttranslational modification and role of HBx. The protein contains three domains from N- to C-terminal region: an oligomerization domain (OD; aa 21-50); a mitochondria association domain (MT; aa 68-104), which is essential for cell death but not for transactivation function; and a transactivation domain (TAD; aa 132-140). Five posttranslational modifications have been described so far (Serines 31, 39, 41, 43 and 75) involving PKC and MAPK pathways. Moreover, HBx displays two independent pro-oncogenic and pro-apoptotic domains that allow it to modulate cell cycle, DNA repair, HBV replication, transcription, apoptosis and cell adhesion. HBx has been shown to interact with several cellular proteins like p53 in its C-terminal region. Even if its localization is still a matter of debate, HBx may be found in the mitochondria or in the nucleus and/or in the cytoplasm depending to its concentration.

As a multifunctional protein exhibiting numerous activities, HBx may be referred as "*the super-HBV gangster in HCC*". Indeed, it affects gene transcription, intracellular signal transduction, cell proliferation, apoptotic cell death and DNA repair (Figure 2) and any or all of these activities could contribute to HCC. The localization of HBx remains a matter of debate. Some studies demonstrated its localization in the cytoplasm or in the mitochondria, whereas others found the protein preferentially in the nucleus, or present in both the cytoplasm and the nucleus [11-14]. As a possible explanation to these contradictory findings, other studies from different laboratories have shown that HBx expressed at very low level is predominantly nuclear, whereas high levels of expression lead to a cytoplasmic accumulation [15, 16].

Overall, it seems that there is a dual localization of HBx: during virus replication, HBx could fluctuate depending on its concentration, but also on the accessibility of cellular partners involved in its nuclear import and export. Its cellular partners will be developed in the next part of this chapter.

Influence of Genotypes

Eight genotypes (A through H) of HBV have been identified that differ from each other in whole-genome sequencing by at least 8% [17-21]. In addition, the major HBV genotypes apart from E and H have been divided into subgenotypes (1, 2, 3, etc.) based on phylogenetic analyses and genetic divergence of complete genomes.

Genotype A is common in North-Western Europe, North America, and Africa. Genotypes B and C are predominant in East and South-East Asia, Oceania and among aboriginal populations in Australia. Genotype D is found worldwide and is predominant in the Mediterranean, Middle East, and India, whereas genotype E has been so far confined to populations in western parts of sub-Saharan Africa apart from one report from India [22, 23].

Genotype G has been identified in samples from several countries, and is found in patients co-infected with another HBV genotype. Genotypes F and H are found mainly in Central and South America, and are the indigenous genotypes of Amerindian populations [17, 22, 24, 25].

Several studies analyzed the outcomes of HBV infection in relation to specific infecting HBV genotypes. Genotype A1 is associated with HCC in young men who are usually and anti-HBe–positive, have low levels of HBV DNA, and rarely display cirrhosis, while genotype A2 is associated with HCC in older persons. Compared to genotype D, genotype A2 is associated with a lower risk of HCC and has a greater resolution of active hepatitis [26].

Table 1. Association between HBV genotypes and disease outcomes

Geno-type	Geographic Region	Disease Association
A1	Sub-Saharan Africa	HCC in young males often without cirrhosis
A2	Northern Europe	HCC and cirrhosis in older persons
B1	Japan	HCC and cirrhosis in older persons
B2-6	East Asia	HCC and cirrhosis occur at younger age than B1
C	China, Korea, South-East Asia, Japan, South Pacific Islands	Higher risk of HCC and cirrhosis compared with genotypes B, A, D and F1
D1-4	Russia, Middle East, Mediterranean, North Africa, Eastern Europe, Indian Subcontinent	Anti-HBe chronic hepatitis B, HCC, and cirrhosis in older individuals
F1	Alaska, Central America, South America	HCC in children and young adults in Alaska only

A study from India reported that genotype D was associated with more severe liver disease and HCC in younger patients than genotype A [27].Most of the current knowledge is based on studies of Asian patients which are infected principally by genotypes B and C. Genotype B causes a shorter duration of high levels of HBV replication with spontaneous HBeAg seroconversion and therefore results in less active liver disease. Genotype B-associated HCC was found primarily in persons older than 60 years. In most of the studies, genotype C has been associated with an increased risk of HCC and HBeAg seroconversion occurs 10-30 years later than genotypes A, B, D, and F1. Genotype C-associated HCC occurred in significantly younger persons ($\leq$50 years) [26, 28-31]. Genotype F1 is associated with HCC in Alaskan natives. Certain HBV genotypes and subgenotypes, including genotypes C, B2-5, and F1, appear to be associated with a higher risk of developing HCC, and others, including genotypes B1, B6, and A2, appear to be associated with a lower risk of complications of HBV (Table 1) [26]. Finally, treatment responses to interferon-α apparently vary according to the viral genotype, infections with strains A and B responding better than those due to genotype C or D.

Genetic Mechanisms of HCC

Genetic mechanisms are involved in the development of HCC: HBV integration into the host genome induces genetic instability and viral proteins encoded by integrated sequences act as trans-activating factors of cellular pathways.

HBV Integration

During the course of HBV chronic infection, viral DNA integration can occur into the host genome. This event is not essential for the viral replication but would allow the persistence of the viral genome in the liver. Integration of HBV DNA into the host genome is found in 85–90% of HBV-related HCCs [32]. Moreover this would occur early before HCC appearance as some integration events were observed in the liver of patients suffering from acute and active chronic hepatitis [33, 34]. Whether the integration occurs randomly into the host genome is still a matter of debate. Several significant sites have been described, like *hTERT* [35-38], the chromosome 17 containing *TP53* [39-41], and the chromosome 3 [33]. However, no specific genes have been identified so far to be a preferential target for HBV insertion, unlike for the woodchuck hepatitis B virus (WHV), which preferentially inserts its DNA genome into *c-Myc* or *N-Myc* genes in the woodchuck genome.

Viral genome insertions are shown to be facilitated by cellular conditions that disrupt host genomic stability or increase cellular DNA replication, such as exposure to oxidative stress or DNA-damaging agents, deficiency of the DNA repair machinery, co-infection with other viruses and chronic liver injuries that increase hepatocyte turnover [32].

Genetic Instability

The insertion itself can induce general genetic instability in host cells: integrated viral sequences are often characterized by rearrangements and/or partial deletions and HBV integration can also induce deletions in the host genome at the integration site. For example, a deletion of 2285 base pairs (bp) in the promoter region of *hTERT* and a deletion of 863 bp in HBV integrated sequence have been reported in one HCC case [35].

HBV Integration Exerts a *cis* Effect

Most of HCC cases contain one or several copies of integrated viral DNA [38]. Numerous studies analyzing the integration profile of HBV DNA in human tumors have shown a clonal proliferation of cells with the same integration site. Many of integration sites are located in or near genes involved in cellular signal pathways or playing key cellular functions (Table 2). Thus integration itself could exert a *cis* effect by deregulating important cellular components.

In one study, HBV integration was observed in the intron 2 of the gene encoding Cyclin A, leading to the synthesis of a chimeric protein Cyclin A – HBV by using the viral promoter PreS2/S [44]. This protein was stabilized as the N-terminus of Cyclin A was truncated and replaced by PreS2/S sequences. In the cell line Huh4 which is derived from a HCC, a viral integration was observed in the promoter region of *hTERT* [37]: transcription occurred through viral and endogen promoters; moreover HBV enhancer sequence was located at about 1.6kb upstream the initiation site of transcription leading to a *cis* activation.

Table 2. HBV integration sites and signaling pathways

Pathways	Genes	References
Ras	*IRAK2, MAPK1*	[38]
Calcium	*SERCA1*	[36]
	NTRK2, IP3R1, IP3R2	[38]
Transcription	*TRAP150*a	[36]
	TRUP, EMX2-like	[38]
	RARb	[42]
Cell cycle	*cyclin A*	[43, 44]
	NMP84p	[36]
DNA replication	*MCM8*	[36]
	hTERT	[35-38]

Taken together, though the insertion of HBV DNA into the host genome might be a random event, it contributes to the formation of an unstable environment, and occasionally induces genomic alterations that may facilitate hepatocyte transformation. Therefore, HBV integration may contribute, at least in part, to the development of most of HBV-induced HCCs.

HBV Integration Exerts a Trans-Activation Effect

In most integrated subviral HBV genomes, the ORF for HBx or Pre-S2 regulatory protein is conserved and can be transcribed [45]. These proteins are transcriptional transactivators and are known to be involved in liver cell proliferation and hepatocarcinogenesis. A category of pre-S2 activators has been described and corresponds to pre-S/S 3'-truncated sequences [45, 46]. These sequences encode C-terminally truncated M (M^t) surface proteins that display a regulatory protein function. This truncation induces modification in the conformation of this M^t protein and allows the pre-S2 region to interact with cytosolic proteins and to activate signaling pathways in the host cell. L proteins can play a role in *trans*-activation as well. Indeed, they display a topology where their pre-S region is entirely directed into the cytoplasm. Truncated L mutants have also been described. These pre-S2 activators activate and interact directly with PKC-α, which results in the phosphorylation of the pre-S2 domain. This activation induces the c-Raf-1/MEK/ERK cascade that favors tumor progression [47, 48]. Transgenic mice for M^t protein developed liver tumors after 10 months. In addition, transgenic mice for L protein developed liver tumors as well [49]. In that case, the overexpression of L protein induces a permanent inflammation that would lead to tumorigenesis. Thus, the regulatory function of L protein would be a supplemental factor favoring the tumor development in mice: protein accumulation due to the stress and inflammation result in critical mutations, and the permanent activation of the c-Raf-1/MEK/ERK pathway in parallel favors tumorigenesis. Moreover, ΔS2-L mutants can positively regulate cyclin A expression and induce cell cycle progression [50].

HBx is also a *trans*-activator of several genes *in vitro*, among which oncogenes like *MYC* [51], *JUN* [52] and *FOS* [53], which would favor the development of HCC [54], and *FAK* that could favor migration and cellular invasion [55]. Furthermore, HBx could inhibit apoptosis induced by p53, TNF, Fas or TGF-beta, while it was shown to promote cell death by inducing mitochondrial aggregation and cytochrome c release (Figure 2) or by sensitizing cells to TNF. Moreover, HBx interacts with DDB1 (UV-damaged DNA-binding protein 1), which plays a role in DNA repair and in cell cycle regulation. Through this interaction, HBx interferes with cell cycle progression into S-phase and induces lagging chromosomes during mitosis [56]. This effect may cause cell proliferation to slow down, and at the same time may create a form of genetic instability contributing to cancer. Studies on the role of HBx have shown that HBx is often accompanied by the loss of C-terminus domain, the full-length protein being detectable in only about 20% of HCC cases with integrated HBx. They have shown that truncated HBx protein can be produced and many 3'-truncated *HBX* gene products retain the transactivation function. In a recent study, Ma and collaborators have shown that transfection of a truncated form of HBx (lacking the p53 interaction domain) increased cell proliferation, whereas transfection of full length HBx had an anti-proliferative, pro-apoptotic effect [57]. While some studies concluded that COOH-truncated HBx proteins retain transcriptional transactivation ability, others found that they have lost most of the activities associated with wild-type HBx, in particular that they can enhance (instead of inhibit) the transforming activity of Ras and Myc [58]. It is possible that the *HBX* gene used in these experiments as well as the lifelong expression of HBx could impact on the development of HCC. However, even if further studies are needed to confirm that HBx can directly induce transformation in mice, its role as a cofactor of carcinogenesis is well accepted.

Occult HBV Infections

Prevalence of Occult HBV and HCC

Chronic HBV infection is one of the main factors for the development of fibrosis, cirrhosis and HCC worldwide. This infection is characterized by the presence for more than 6 months of HBsAg and HBV DNA. Thanks to the improvement of detection tools for HBV since the 80's, occult HBV infections (OBI) were described. OBI is defined by the presence of HBV DNA in the liver tissue and/or in the serum of HBsAg-negative patients associated usually with a low HBV viremia (10^1 to 10^4 copies/ml).

Two types of OBI can be distinguished: (i) seropositive OBI with the presence of HBV DNA in the liver and/or in the serum with anti-HBs and/or anti-HBc seroconversion, and (ii) seronegative OBI characterized by the presence of HBV DNA in the liver and/or in the serum in the absence of anti-HBs and HBc seroconversion [59]. The prevalence of OBI worldwide is not clear due to the different sensitivity and specificity of the methods used for detection [60]. An Italian study concerning people without liver disease revealed OBI in 16.3% of the population and in association with anti-HBc positive status [61]. However, in a Korean study concerning healthy adults, OBI was found in 0.7% of the population [62]. OBI was also investigated among chronic hepatitis patients with unknown etiology. In a cohort of 50 HBsAg-negative patients with non-A non-C non-E hepatitis, OBI was present in 30% of the cases and responsible for liver lesions [63]. In an HBsAg-negative hemophilia Japanese cohort in which a high prevalence of infection with transfusion-transmissible agents occurred, 51.2% of patients were positive for OBI [64]. OBI is usually characterized by a low level HBV replication leading to low viremia. However, in particular context OBI can reactivate and a high HBV viremia can be observed. Such cases of reactivations occur mostly with an immune-depressive status induced by therapies and/or related to diseases that involve the immune system [65]. OBI is the consequence of the persistence of cccDNA in the nucleus of hepatocytes [66]. Most of patients with OBI are infected with replication competent virus showing a suppression of replication and gene expression. OBI may be explained by the appearance of mutations in the immunodominant loop of HBV surface antigen, thus altering HBsAg antigenicity, or the suppression of viral replication due to (i) mutations in the viral polymerase or (ii) virus-host interactions and epigenetic factors [67].

Occult strains usually persist as free episomal forms which are transcriptionnally active, thus maintaining (i) a chronic liver inflammation, (ii) the tumorigenic properties of the virus *via* HBx protein, and (iii) a potential viral integration in the host genome, leading to hepatoma transformation [68]. To understand the implication of OBI in HCC development, an Italian team analyzed in HCC patients with OBI the molecular and functional aspects of the HBV strains involved.

It appeared clearly that HBV strains are *in vitro* replication competent without harboring any mutation that could be responsible for an *in vivo* inhibition of HBV replication [69]. This study underlines the fact that HBV strains in OBI are replication competent and by this way can exert also, with a low level of HBV replication, the oncogenic potential of the virus. Experiments in animal models demonstrated that woodchucks, once infected with WHV, are at risk of developing HCC even after the 'apparent' clearance of the virus [70].

In this context, a retrospective cohort of cirrhotic patients without overt HCV or HBV infection were screened for the presence of HBV DNA (C and X genes) by sensitive PCR. The carcinogenesis rates related to OBI were investigated in two groups, HBV DNA-positive group and HBV DNA-negative group: the rates were 27.0% and 11.8% after 5 year, and 100% and 17.6% after 10 years, respectively. Therefore the presence of HBV DNA in the cirrhotic liver increased the risk of HCC development by 8, demonstrating a clear correlation between OBI and HCC in cirrhotic patients [71].

HBV and HCV Co-infection

Hepatitis C virus (HCV) is a member of the *flaviviridae* family, which affects 130 million people worldwide and is responsible for cirrhosis, fibrosis and HCC. This virus is mainly transmitted by blood products and drug injection. It is estimated that 7 to 20 million people are co-infected by HBV/HCV worldwide with a higher prevalence in HBV endemic regions (Asia, South America and Sub-Saharian Africa). In areas with a low prevalence for HBsAg (< 1% for example in Europe), HBV/HCV co-infection is considered as very rare.

HBV and HCV have little in common during their life cycle except their preferential replication in the same target organ: the liver. HBV/HCV co-infection is associated with a more severe liver disease, a faster development of HCC and a higher mortality rate compared with HBV or HCV mono-infection [72]. Several studies have shown that HBV/HCV co-infected patients have lower levels of HBV DNA, associated with a decreased activity of HBV polymerase and a diminution of HBsAg and HBcAg in the liver. During co-infection HCV seems to have a dominant effect leading to the suppression of HBV replication.

Little is known about the molecular mechanism of inhibition of HBV during co-infection with HCV: *in vitro* studies suggest a suppression of HBV DNA transcription by the hepatitis C core protein [73, 74]. However another study observed an inhibition of HCV by active HBV replication in chronic carriers [75]. Nothing indicates a direct interaction between both viruses and it was proposed that molecular indirect effects of host-viral interactions may be responsible for a dual inhibition [76-78].

It is to notice that HCV infected patients are a population with a high rate of OBI. HBV DNA is detectable in one third of HBsAg-negative HCV carriers in the Mediterranean basin [79] and the prevalence seems to be higher in East Asian countries. Studies made in the Japanese population reported a prevalence between 37% and 95 % [80].

Another study reported a prevalence of 43.6% in HCV-positive patients for whom the degree of inflammatory cell infiltration and irregular regeneration of hepatocytes was significantly greater than for HBV DNA-negative patients [81]. Furthermore the probability for developing HCC was significantly higher in HBV DNA-positive patients (76.3%) than in HBV DNA-negative patients (23.7%). Finally OBI in co-infection with HCV is responsible for advanced liver fibrosis and HCC development [81, 82].

HBV and HIV Co-infection

Human immunodeficiency virus (HIV) is a member of the lentivirus family affecting 40 million people worldwide and responsible for the Acquired Immune Deficiency Syndrome. It shares the same routes of transmission as HBV (sexual, blood transfusion, mother-to-child), leading to a high frequency of co-infections: it is estimated that 2-4 million HIV-positive individuals are chronically infected with HBV [83]. With the introduction of highly active anti-retroviral treatment (HAART) to cure HIV, HIV infection is considered as a chronic disease and hepatic disease due to HBV or HCV is one of the first causes of morbidity and mortality in HIV-positive patients [84]. Furthermore drugs used to treat HIV, principally lamivudine, are also active against HBV and may increase the risk of drug-related hepato-toxicity and impact on the selection of drug-resistant HBV mutants and escape mutants. During HBV/HIV co-infection HBV does not seem to affect HIV disease but the opposite is not true. Some studies reported a higher rate of HBV chronicity than during HBV mono-infection [85], a higher level of HBV replication, a lower rate of spontaneous loss of HBeAg and/or HBsAg, and a lower anti-HBs and anti-HBe seroconversion.

Importantly, progression to fibrosis, cirrhosis and HCC is faster than during HBV mono-infection [86]. In HIV-positive patients, OBI is correlated with anti-HBc seroconversion status and HCV triple co-infection. In a HIV(+), HBsAg(-), anti-HBc(+) cohort, 15% of patients were positive for HBV DNA with a clear correlation between OBI and HCV positivity: 21% *versus* 8% for HCV(-) individuals [87].

In a HIV(+) Brazilian cohort, OBI was found in 14% (6/43) of patients in association with a HCV(+) status, a low HBV viral load but not with alanine aminotransferase (ALT) elevated levels. HBV strains were isolated by a molecular analysis from HIV-positive patients treated by HAART and HBV strains harboring modifications were identified: one modification in the S gene that can affect antigenicity, and another in the P gene conferring drug resistance [88].

Interestingly, the strain harboring drug resistance mutations displayed a low viremia. This underlines the multi-factorial mechanism of OBI. Actually, it is clear that in HIV-positive patients, one of the first risks associated with OBI is the selection and reactivation of HBV resistant strains or escape mutants due to a cessation of HAART treatment or an immunosuppressive status [88, 89], thus complicating clinical treatment and increasing liver damage.

Conclusion

Since the late 1980s many studies have been carried out on occult HBV. The detection of OBI in patients with chronic hepatitis in association or not with different risk factors such as HCV or alcohol abuse may identify individuals at higher risk of progression toward cirrhosis and possibly HCC. OBI detection may be recommended in patients undergoing chemotherapy and/or immunosuppressive treatments and most importantly blood and organ donors to undergo preventive treatment with antivirals.

Unfortunately, until now, there is no standard method to detect OBI: the 'Statements from the Taormina expert meeting on occult hepatitis B virus infection' suggested to use the same oligonucleotide primers for detection of occult HBV DNA through 'nested' PCR amplification. The possible use of standardized tools for OBI detection is very interesting in terms of harmonization of all data to compare studies. Furthermore, it is clear in terms of OBI infection that searching anti-HBs/anti-HBc is not a discriminatory test. The development of molecular tests (HBV DNA) may be an important step towards a better understanding and detection of this type of infection.

References

[1] Glebe Dand Urban S, Viral and cellular determinants involved in hepadnaviral entry, *World J. Gastroenterol.*, 2007 Jan 7, 13 (1), 22-38.
[2] Leistner CM, Gruen-Bernhard Sand Glebe D, Role of glycosaminoglycans for binding and infection of hepatitis B virus, *Cell Microbiol*, 2008 Jan, 10 (1), 122-33.
[3] Kann M, Schmitz Aand Rabe B, Intracellular transport of hepatitis B virus, *World J. Gastroenterol.*, 2007 Jan 7, 13 (1), 39-47.
[4] Hu Jand Lin L, RNA-protein interactions in hepadnavirus reverse transcription, *Front Biosci.*, 2009, 14, 1606-18.

[5] Summers Jand Mason WS, Replication of the genome of a hepatitis B--like virus by reverse transcription of an RNA intermediate, *Cell*, 1982 Jun, 29 (2), 403-15.

[6] Patient R, Hourioux Cand Roingeard P, Morphogenesis of hepatitis B virus and its subviral envelope particles, *Cell Microbiol.*, 2009 Nov, 11 (11), 1561-70.

[7] Glebe D, Recent advances in hepatitis B virus research: a German point of view, *World J. Gastroenterol.*, 2007 Jan 7, 13 (1), 8-13.

[8] Hsieh YH, Su IJ, Wang HC, Chang WW, Lei HY, Lai MD, Chang WTand Huang W, Pre-S mutant surface antigens in chronic hepatitis B virus infection induce oxidative stress and DNA damage, *Carcinogenesis*, 2004 Oct, 25 (10), 2023-32.

[9] Gunther S, Fischer L, Pult I, Sterneck Mand Will H, Naturally occurring variants of hepatitis B virus, *Adv. Virus Res.*, 1999, 52, 25-137.

[10] Fan YF, Lu CC, Chen WC, Yao WJ, Wang HC, Chang TT, Lei HY, Shiau ALand Su IJ, Prevalence and significance of hepatitis B virus (HBV) pre-S mutants in serum and liver at different replicative stages of chronic HBV infection, *Hepatology*, 2001 Jan, 33 (1), 277-86.

[11] Doria M, Klein N, Lucito Rand Schneider RJ, The hepatitis B virus HBx protein is a dual specificity cytoplasmic activator of Ras and nuclear activator of transcription factors, *EMBO J.*, 1995 Oct 2, 14 (19), 4747-57.

[12] Schek N, Bartenschlager R, Kuhn Cand Schaller H, Phosphorylation and rapid turnover of hepatitis B virus X-protein expressed in HepG2 cells from a recombinant vaccinia virus, *Oncogene*, 1991 Oct, 6 (10), 1735-44.

[13] Sirma H, Weil R, Rosmorduc O, Urban S, Israel A, Kremsdorf Dand Brechot C, Cytosol is the prime compartment of hepatitis B virus X protein where it colocalizes with the proteasome, *Oncogene*, 1998 Apr 23, 16 (16), 2051-63.

[14] Weil R, Sirma H, Giannini C, Kremsdorf D, Bessia C, Dargemont C, Brechot Cand Israel A, Direct association and nuclear import of the hepatitis B virus X protein with the NF-kappaB inhibitor IkappaBalpha, *Mol. Cell Biol.*, 1999 Sep, 19 (9), 6345-54.

[15] Cha MY, Ryu DK, Jung HS, Chang HEand Ryu WS, Stimulation of hepatitis B virus genome replication by HBx is linked to both nuclear and cytoplasmic HBx expression, *J. Gen. Virol.*, 2009 Apr, 90 (Pt 4), 978-86.

[16] Henkler F, Hoare J, Waseem N, Goldin RD, McGarvey MJ, Koshy Rand King IA, Intracellular localization of the hepatitis B virus HBx protein, *J. Gen. Virol.*, 2001 Apr, 82 (Pt 4), 871-82.
[17] Arauz-Ruiz P, Norder H, Robertson BHand Magnius LO, Genotype H: a new Amerindian genotype of hepatitis B virus revealed in Central America, *J. Gen. Virol.*, 2002 Aug, 83 (Pt 8), 2059-73.
[18] Naumann H, Schaefer S, Yoshida CF, Gaspar AM, Repp Rand Gerlich WH, Identification of a new hepatitis B virus (HBV) genotype from Brazil that expresses HBV surface antigen subtype adw4, *J. Gen. Virol.*, 1993 Aug, 74 (Pt 8), 1627-32.
[19] Norder H, Courouce AMand Magnius LO, Complete genomes, phylogenetic relatedness, and structural proteins of six strains of the hepatitis B virus, four of which represent two new genotypes, *Virology*, 1994 Feb, 198 (2), 489-503.
[20] Okamoto H, Imai M, Tsuda F, Tanaka T, Miyakawa Yand Mayumi M, Point mutation in the S gene of hepatitis B virus for a d/y or w/r subtypic change in two blood donors carrying a surface antigen of compound subtype adyr or adwr, *J. Virol.*, 1987 Oct, 61 (10), 3030-4.
[21] Stuyver L, De Gendt S, Van Geyt C, Zoulim F, Fried M, Schinazi RFand Rossau R, A new genotype of hepatitis B virus: complete genome and phylogenetic relatedness, *J. Gen. Virol.*, 2000 Jan, 81 (Pt 1), 67-74.
[22] Norder H, Courouce AM, Coursaget P, Echevarria JM, Lee SD, Mushahwar IK, Robertson BH, Locarnini Sand Magnius LO, Genetic diversity of hepatitis B virus strains derived worldwide: genotypes, subgenotypes, and HBsAg subtypes, *Intervirology*, 2004 Nov-Dec, 47 (6), 289-309.
[23] Singh J, Dickens C, Pahal V, Kumar R, Chaudhary R, Kramvis Aand Kew MC, First report of genotype e of hepatitis B virus in an Indian population, *Intervirology*, 2009, 52 (5), 235-8.
[24] Kumagai I, Abe K, Oikawa T, Sato A, Sato S, Endo R, Takikawa Y, Suzuki K, Masuda T, Sainokami S, Endo K, Takahashi Mand Okamoto H, A male patient with severe acute hepatitis who was domestically infected with a genotype H hepatitis B virus in Iwate, Japan, *J. Gastroenterol.*, 2007 Feb, 42 (2), 168-75.
[25] Sanchez LV, Tanaka Y, Maldonado M, Mizokami Mand Panduro A, Difference of hepatitis B virus genotype distribution in two groups of mexican patients with different risk factors. High prevalence of genotype H and G, *Intervirology*, 2007, 50 (1), 9-15.

[26] McMahon BJ, The influence of hepatitis B virus genotype and subgenotype on the natural history of chronic hepatitis B, *Hepatol. Int.*, 2009 Jun, 3 (2), 334-42.
[27] Thakur V, Guptan RC, Kazim SN, Malhotra Vand Sarin SK, Profile, spectrum and significance of HBV genotypes in chronic liver disease patients in the Indian subcontinent, *J. Gastroenterol. Hepatol.*, 2002 Feb, 17 (2), 165-70.
[28] Kao JH, Hepatitis B virus genotypes and hepatocellular carcinoma in Taiwan, *Intervirology*, 2003, 46 (6), 400-7.
[29] Kao JH, Chen PJ, Lai MYand Chen DS, Hepatitis B genotypes correlate with clinical outcomes in patients with chronic hepatitis B, *Gastroenterology*, 2000 Mar, 118 (3), 554-9.
[30] Lee CM, Chen CH, Lu SN, Tung HD, Chou WJ, Wang JH, Chen TM, Hung CH, Huang CCand Chen WJ, Prevalence and clinical implications of hepatitis B virus genotypes in southern Taiwan, *Scand. J. Gastroenterol.*, 2003 Jan, 38 (1), 95-101.
[31] Tangkijvanich P, Mahachai V, Komolmit P, Fongsarun J, Theamboonlers Aand Poovorawan Y, Hepatitis B virus genotypes and hepatocellular carcinoma in Thailand, *World J. Gastroenterol.*, 2005 Apr 21, 11 (15), 2238-43.
[32] Bonilla Guerrero Rand Roberts LR, The role of hepatitis B virus integrations in the pathogenesis of human hepatocellular carcinoma, *J. Hepatol.*, 2005 May, 42 (5), 760-77.
[33] Minami M, Daimon Y, Mori K, Takashima H, Nakajima T, Itoh Yand Okanoue T, Hepatitis B virus-related insertional mutagenesis in chronic hepatitis B patients as an early drastic genetic change leading to hepatocarcinogenesis, *Oncogene*, 2005 Jun 23, 24 (27), 4340-8.
[34] Murakami Y, Minami M, Daimon Yand Okanoue T, Hepatitis B virus DNA in liver, serum, and peripheral blood mononuclear cells after the clearance of serum hepatitis B virus surface antigen, *J. Med. Virol.*, 2004 Feb, 72 (2), 203-14.
[35] Ferber MJ, Montoya DP, Yu C, Aderca I, McGee A, Thorland EC, Nagorney DM, Gostout BS, Burgart LJ, Boix L, Bruix J, McMahon BJ, Cheung TH, Chung TK, Wong YF, Smith DIand Roberts LR, Integrations of the hepatitis B virus (HBV) and human papillomavirus (HPV) into the human telomerase reverse transcriptase (hTERT) gene in liver and cervical cancers, *Oncogene*, 2003 Jun 12, 22 (24), 3813-20.

[36] Gozuacik D, Murakami Y, Saigo K, Chami M, Mugnier C, Lagorce D, Okanoue T, Urashima T, Brechot Cand Paterlini-Brechot P, Identification of human cancer-related genes by naturally occurring Hepatitis B Virus DNA tagging, *Oncogene*, 2001 Sep 27, 20 (43), 6233-40.
[37] Horikawa Iand Barrett JC, cis-Activation of the human telomerase gene (hTERT) by the hepatitis B virus genome, *J. Natl. Cancer Inst.*, 2001 Aug 1, 93 (15), 1171-3.
[38] Paterlini-Brechot P, Saigo K, Murakami Y, Chami M, Gozuacik D, Mugnier C, Lagorce Dand Brechot C, Hepatitis B virus-related insertional mutagenesis occurs frequently in human liver cancers and recurrently targets human telomerase gene, *Oncogene*, 2003 Jun 19, 22 (25), 3911-6.
[39] Liu XH, Lin J, Zhang SH, Zhang SM, Feitelson MA, Gao HJand Zhu MH, COOH-terminal deletion of HBx gene is a frequent event in HBV-associated hepatocellular carcinoma, *World J. Gastroenterol.*, 2008 Mar 7, 14 (9), 1346-52.
[40] Slagle BL, Zhou YZand Butel JS, Hepatitis B virus integration event in human chromosome 17p near the p53 gene identifies the region of the chromosome commonly deleted in virus-positive hepatocellular carcinomas, *Cancer Res.*, 1991 Jan 1, 51 (1), 49-54.
[41] Zhou YZ, Slagle BL, Donehower LA, vanTuinen P, Ledbetter DHand Butel JS, Structural analysis of a hepatitis B virus genome integrated into chromosome 17p of a human hepatocellular carcinoma, *J. Virol.*, 1988 Nov, 62 (11), 4224-31.
[42] Dejean A, Bougueleret L, Grzeschik KHand Tiollais P, Hepatitis B virus DNA integration in a sequence homologous to v-erb-A and steroid receptor genes in a hepatocellular carcinoma, *Nature*, 1986 Jul 3-9, 322 (6074), 70-2.
[43] Wang J, Chenivesse X, Henglein Band Brechot C, Hepatitis B virus integration in a cyclin A gene in a hepatocellular carcinoma, *Nature*, 1990 Feb 8, 343 (6258), 555-7.
[44] Wang J, Zindy F, Chenivesse X, Lamas E, Henglein Band Brechot C, Modification of cyclin A expression by hepatitis B virus DNA integration in a hepatocellular carcinoma, *Oncogene*, 1992 Aug, 7 (8), 1653-6.

[45] Schluter V, Meyer M, Hofschneider PH, Koshy Rand Caselmann WH, Integrated hepatitis B virus X and 3' truncated preS/S sequences derived from human hepatomas encode functionally active transactivators, *Oncogene*, 1994 Nov, 9 (11), 3335-44.

[46] Lupberger Jand Hildt E, Hepatitis B virus-induced oncogenesis, *World J. Gastroenterol.*, 2007 Jan 7, 13 (1), 74-81.

[47] Hildt E, Munz B, Saher G, Reifenberg Kand Hofschneider PH, The PreS2 activator MHBs(t) of hepatitis B virus activates c-raf-1/Erk2 signaling in transgenic mice, *EMBO J.*, 2002 Feb 15, 21 (4), 525-35.

[48] Hildt E, Saher G, Bruss Vand Hofschneider PH, The hepatitis B virus large surface protein (LHBs) is a transcriptional activator, *Virology*, 1996 Nov 1, 225 (1), 235-9.

[49] Chisari FV, Klopchin K, Moriyama T, Pasquinelli C, Dunsford HA, Sell S, Pinkert CA, Brinster RLand Palmiter RD, Molecular pathogenesis of hepatocellular carcinoma in hepatitis B virus transgenic mice, *Cell*, 1989 Dec 22, 59 (6), 1145-56.

[50] Wang HC, Chang WT, Chang WW, Wu HC, Huang W, Lei HY, Lai MD, Fausto Nand Su IJ, Hepatitis B virus pre-S2 mutant upregulates cyclin A expression and induces nodular proliferation of hepatocytes, *Hepatology*, 2005 Apr, 41 (4), 761-70.

[51] Balsano C, Avantaggiati ML, Natoli G, De Marzio E, Will H, Perricaudet Mand Levrero M, Full-length and truncated versions of the hepatitis B virus (HBV) X protein (pX) transactivate the cmyc protooncogene at the transcriptional level, *Biochem. Biophys. Res. Commun.*, 1991 May 15, 176 (3), 985-92.

[52] Twu JS, Lai MY, Chen DSand Robinson WS, Activation of protooncogene c-jun by the X protein of hepatitis B virus, *Virology*, 1993 Jan, 192 (1), 346-50.

[53] Avantaggiati ML, Natoli G, Balsano C, Chirillo P, Artini M, De Marzio E, Collepardo Dand Levrero M, The hepatitis B virus (HBV) pX transactivates the c-fos promoter through multiple cis-acting elements, *Oncogene*, 1993 Jun, 8 (6), 1567-74.

[54] Diao J, Garces Rand Richardson CD, X protein of hepatitis B virus modulates cytokine and growth factor related signal transduction pathways during the course of viral infections and hepatocarcinogenesis, *Cytokine Growth Factor Rev.*, 2001 Jun-Sep, 12 (2-3), 189-205.

[55] Bouchard MJ, Wang Land Schneider RJ, Activation of focal adhesion kinase by hepatitis B virus HBx protein: multiple functions in viral replication, *J. Virol.*, 2006 May, 80 (9), 4406-14.

[56] Martin-Lluesma S, Schaeffer C, Robert EI, van Breugel PC, Leupin O, Hantz Oand Strubin M, Hepatitis B virus X protein affects S phase progression leading to chromosome segregation defects by binding to damaged DNA binding protein 1, *Hepatology*, 2008 Nov, 48 (5), 1467-76.
[57] Ma NF, Lau SH, Hu L, Xie D, Wu J, Yang J, Wang Y, Wu MC, Fung J, Bai X, Tzang CH, Fu L, Yang M, Su YAand Guan XY, COOH-terminal truncated HBV X protein plays key role in hepatocarcinogenesis, *Clin. Cancer Res.*, 2008 Aug 15, 14 (16), 5061-8.
[58] Tu H, Bonura C, Giannini C, Mouly H, Soussan P, Kew M, Paterlini-Brechot P, Brechot Cand Kremsdorf D, Biological impact of natural COOH-terminal deletions of hepatitis B virus X protein in hepatocellular carcinoma tissues, *Cancer Res.*, 2001 Nov 1, 61 (21), 7803-10.
[59] Raimondo G, Allain JP, Brunetto MR, Buendia MA, Chen DS, Colombo M, Craxi A, Donato F, Ferrari C, Gaeta GB, Gerlich WH, Levrero M, Locarnini S, Michalak T, Mondelli MU, Pawlotsky JM, Pollicino T, Prati D, Puoti M, Samuel D, Shouval D, Smedile A, Squadrito G, Trepo C, Villa E, Will H, Zanetti ARand Zoulim F, Statements from the Taormina expert meeting on occult hepatitis B virus infection, *J. Hepatol.*, 2008 Oct, 49 (4), 652-7.
[60] Torbenson Mand Thomas DL, Occult hepatitis B, *Lancet Infect. Dis.*, 2002 Aug, 2 (8), 479-86.
[61] Raimondo G, Navarra G, Mondello S, Costantino L, Colloredo G, Cucinotta E, Di Vita G, Scisca C, Squadrito Gand Pollicino T, Occult hepatitis B virus in liver tissue of individuals without hepatic disease, *J. Hepatol.*, 2008 May, 48 (5), 743-6.
[62] Song EY, Yun YM, Park MHand Seo DH, Prevalence of occult hepatitis B virus infection in a general adult population in Korea, *Intervirology*, 2009, 52 (2), 57-62.
[63] Chemin I, Zoulim F, Merle P, Arkhis A, Chevallier M, Kay A, Cova L, Chevallier P, Mandrand Band Trepo C, High incidence of hepatitis B infections among chronic hepatitis cases of unknown aetiology, *J. Hepatol.*, 2001 Mar, 34 (3), 447-54.
[64] Toyoda H, Hayashi K, Murakami Y, Honda T, Katano Y, Nakano I, Goto H, Kumada Tand Takamatsu J, Prevalence and clinical implications of occult hepatitis B viral infection in hemophilia patients in Japan, *J. Med. Virol.*, 2004 Jun, 73 (2), 195-9.

[65] Yeo W, Chan TC, Leung NW, Lam WY, Mo FK, Chu MT, Chan HL, Hui EP, Lei KI, Mok TSand Chan PK, Hepatitis B virus reactivation in lymphoma patients with prior resolved hepatitis B undergoing anticancer therapy with or without rituximab, *J. Clin. Oncol.*, 2009 Feb 1, 27 (4), 605-11.

[66] Zoulim F, New insight on hepatitis B virus persistence from the study of intrahepatic viral cccDNA, *J. Hepatol.*, 2005 Mar, 42 (3), 302-8.

[67] Raimondo G, Pollicino T, Cacciola Iand Squadrito G, Occult hepatitis B virus infection, *J. Hepatol.*, 2007 Jan, 46 (1), 160-70.

[68] Pollicino T, Squadrito G, Cerenzia G, Cacciola I, Raffa G, Craxi A, Farinati F, Missale G, Smedile A, Tiribelli C, Villa Eand Raimondo G, Hepatitis B virus maintains its pro-oncogenic properties in the case of occult HBV infection, *Gastroenterology*, 2004 Jan, 126 (1), 102-10.

[69] Pollicino T, Raffa G, Costantino L, Lisa A, Campello C, Squadrito G, Levrero Mand Raimondo G, Molecular and functional analysis of occult hepatitis B virus isolates from patients with hepatocellular carcinoma, *Hepatology*, 2007 Feb, 45 (2), 277-85.

[70] Korba BE, Wells FV, Baldwin B, Cote PJ, Tennant BC, Popper Hand Gerin JL, Hepatocellular carcinoma in woodchuck hepatitis virus-infected woodchucks: presence of viral DNA in tumor tissue from chronic carriers and animals serologically recovered from acute infections, *Hepatology*, 1989 Mar, 9 (3), 461-70.

[71] Ikeda K, Kobayashi M, Someya T, Saitoh S, Hosaka T, Akuta N, Suzuki F, Suzuki Y, Arase Yand Kumada H, Occult hepatitis B virus infection increases hepatocellular carcinogenesis by eight times in patients with non-B, non-C liver cirrhosis: a cohort study, *J. Viral. Hepat.*, 2009 Jun, 16 (6), 437-43.

[72] Potthoff A, Manns MPand Wedemeyer H, Treatment of HBV/HCV coinfection, *Expert Opin. Pharmacother.*, 2010 Apr, 11 (6), 919-28.

[73] Schuttler CG, Fiedler N, Schmidt K, Repp R, Gerlich WHand Schaefer S, Suppression of hepatitis B virus enhancer 1 and 2 by hepatitis C virus core protein, *J. Hepatol*, 2002 Dec, 37 (6), 855-62.

[74] Shih CM, Lo SJ, Miyamura T, Chen SYand Lee YH, Suppression of hepatitis B virus expression and replication by hepatitis C virus core protein in HuH-7 cells, *J. Virol.*, 1993 Oct, 67 (10), 5823-32.

[75] Pontisso P, Ruvoletto MG, Fattovich G, Chemello L, Gallorini A, Ruol Aand Alberti A, Clinical and virological profiles in patients with multiple hepatitis virus infections, *Gastroenterology*, 1993 Nov, 105 (5), 1529-33.

[76] Bellecave P, Gouttenoire J, Gajer M, Brass V, Koutsoudakis G, Blum HE, Bartenschlager R, Nassal Mand Moradpour D, Hepatitis B and C virus coinfection: a novel model system reveals the absence of direct viral interference, *Hepatology*, 2009 Jul, 50 (1), 46-55.

[77] Eyre NS, Phillips RJ, Bowden S, Yip E, Dewar B, Locarnini SAand Beard MR, Hepatitis B virus and hepatitis C virus interaction in Huh-7 cells, *J. Hepatol.*, 2009 Sep, 51 (3), 446-57.

[78] Koike K, Yasuda K, Yotsuyanagi H, Moriya K, Hino K, Kurokawa Kand Iino S, Dominant replication of either virus in dual infection with hepatitis viruses B and C, *J. Med. Virol.*, 1995 Feb, 45 (2), 236-9.

[79] Cacciola I, Pollicino T, Squadrito G, Cerenzia G, Orlando MEand Raimondo G, Occult hepatitis B virus infection in patients with chronic hepatitis C liver disease, *N. Engl. J. Med.*, 1999 Jul 1, 341 (1), 22-6.

[80] Koike K, Kobayashi M, Gondo M, Hayashi I, Osuga Tand Takada S, Hepatitis B virus DNA is frequently found in liver biopsy samples from hepatitis C virus-infected chronic hepatitis patients, *J. Med. Virol.*, 1998 Apr, 54 (4), 249-55.

[81] Matsuoka S, Nirei K, Tamura A, Nakamura H, Matsumura H, Oshiro S, Arakawa Y, Yamagami H, Tanaka Nand Moriyama M, Influence of occult hepatitis B virus coinfection on the incidence of fibrosis and hepatocellular carcinoma in chronic hepatitis C, *Intervirology*, 2008, 51 (5), 352-61.

[82] Chemin Iand Trepo C, Clinical impact of occult HBV infections, *J. Clin. Virol.*, 2005 Dec, 34 Suppl 1, S15-21.

[83] Alter MJ, Epidemiology of viral hepatitis and HIV co-infection, *J. Hepatol.*, 2006, 44 (1 Suppl), S6-9.

[84] Sulkowski MS, Viral hepatitis and HIV coinfection, *J. Hepatol.*, 2008 Feb, 48 (2), 353-67.

[85] Koblin BA, Taylor PE, Rubinstein Pand Stevens CE, Effect of duration of hepatitis B virus infection on the association between human immunodeficiency virus type-1 and hepatitis B viral replication, *Hepatology*, 1992 Apr, 15 (4), 590-2.

[86] Bonacini M, Interaction between HIV and hepatitis B, *AIDS*, 1997 Nov 15, 11 (14), 1789-90.

[87] Morsica G, Ancarani F, Bagaglio S, Maracci M, Cicconi P, Cozzi Lepri A, Antonucci G, Bruno R, Santantonio T, Tacconi L, Baldelli F, Piscopo R, Santoro D, Lazzarin Aand D'Arminio Monforte A, Occult hepatitis B virus infection in a cohort of HIV-positive patients: correlation with hepatitis C virus coinfection, virological and immunological features, *Infection*, 2009 Oct, 37 (5), 445-9.
[88] Araujo NM, Branco-Vieira M, Silva AC, Pilotto JH, Grinsztejn B, de Almeida AJ, Trepo Cand Gomes SA, Occult hepatitis B virus infection in HIV-infected patients: Evaluation of biochemical, virological and molecular parameters, *Hepatol. Res.*, 2008 Dec, 38 (12), 1194-203.
[89] Altfeld M, Rockstroh JK, Addo M, Kupfer B, Pult I, Will Hand Spengler U, Reactivation of hepatitis B in a long-term anti-HBs-positive patient with AIDS following lamivudine withdrawal, *J. Hepatol.*, 1998 Aug, 29 (2), 306-9.

In: Hepatitis B: New Research
Editors: J. T. Cox and D. I. Owen
ISBN 978-1-62081-846-6

Chapter VII

Silencing Hepatitis B Virus Replication with Antiviral Pri-Mir Shuttles Generated from Liver-Specific Pol II Promoters

Abdullah Ely and Patrick Arbuthnot*
Antiviral Gene Therapy Research Unit,
Department of Molecular Medicine and Haematology,
University of the Witwatersrand Medical School, WITS, South Africa

Abstract

Chronic infection with hepatitis B virus (HBV) occurs in approximately 6% of the world's population and is often complicated by cirrhosis and hepatocellular carcinoma (HCC). Existing therapy rarely has durable effects and improving treatment to counter the infection remains an important medical priority. Although harnessing the RNA interference (RNAi) pathway to achieve therapeutic HBV gene silencing

* Corresponding author: Tel: +27 (0)11 717 2365; Fax: +27 (0)11 717 2395; E-mail: Patrick.Arbuthnot@wits.ac.za

holds promise, precise regulation of the expression of silencing sequences is critically important for safe application of this approach. Earlier work from our laboratory demonstrated that pri-miR-31- and pri-miR-122-based anti HBV shuttles were capable of potent, safe antiviral activity and can be used in modular multimeric arrangements.

To advance this approach, and limit the potential problems caused by extrahepatic expression of anti HBV RNAi activators, these sequences were placed under control of liver specific transcription control elements, viz. the human Factor VIII (FVIII), alpha-1-antitrypsin (A1AT), HBV preS2 and HBV basic core (BCP) promoters. Using a luciferase reporter gene assay optimal liver-specific transcription control was observed with A1AT and BCP regulating sequences. These elements were then incorporated into pri-miR-expression cassettes and were tested for antiviral efficacy in cell culture and a murine model of HBV replication. Results showed that silencing of HBV replication was achieved. Importantly there was no evidence for disruption of endogenous miR function, which is a significant advantage over use of stronger and constitutively active RNA polymerase (Pol) III promoter RNAi expression cassettes. The use of anti HBV pri-miR shuttles in the context of liver-specific Pol II promoters is likely to have usefulness for therapeutic HBV knockdown, and should also have general applicability to silencing of pathology causing genes in the liver.

Introduction

The hepatitis B virus (HBV) is a human pathogen that infects the liver and causes both acute and chronic disease. An estimated 2 billion people worldwide have been infected with HBV and 350 million individuals are chronic carriers of the virus [1]. Individuals persistently infected with HBV are at an increased risk of developing the severe complications of cirrhosis and hepatocellular carcinoma (HCC) [2]. HCC prognosis is very poor and annual incidence is almost equal to annual mortality [3].

An effective anti HBV vaccine is available and universal vaccination of infants has been implemented in parts of Asia and sub Saharan Africa, where the infection is endemic [4]. Immunization is however prophylactic and offers little therapeutic benefit to existing chronic carriers. Immunomodulators and nucleotide and nucleoside analogues remain the only licensed therapies for management of chronic infections [5].

However current treatment regimens are limited by expense, side effects, development of resistance and efficacy that is not durable. The advancement of novel treatment strategies to limit severe sequelae of chronic HBV infection therefore remains an important medical goal. HBV replication involves reverse transcription of a greater than genome length 3.5 kb pregenomic RNA (pgRNA), which is essential for the formation of partly double stranded relaxed circular DNA (rcDNA) that is typically found in the HB virion (Figure 1A) [6, 7]. After infection of hepatocytes, the rcDNA is converted to a covalently closed circular DNA (cccDNA), which serves as template for transcription of sequences encoding viral proteins and pgRNA.

The viral genome has a highly compact arrangement with overlapping open reading frames (ORFs), which limits its sequence plasticity. Methods that utilize RNA interference (RNAi) to interfere with the stability of pgRNA therefore have the potential to disrupt an essential step of viral replication.

An important consideration in development of RNAi-based therapy for HBV infection is the controlled expression of silencing sequences to avoid potentially harmful unintended effects. Achieving tissue-specific expression of RNAi effecter sequences also mitigates the need for strategies to deliver expression cassettes to target tissues exclusively. We have previously shown that pri-miR-31 or pri-miR-122 may be used as scaffolds for embedding anti HBV guide sequences.

These shuttles could be incorporated into CMV RNA polymerase (Pol) II promoter cassettes and used for efficient knockdown of markers of HBV replication in cultured cells and in vivo [8-10]. Moreover, this approach was used to generate Pol II-expressed multimeric miR shuttles that simultaneously target multiple sites to overcome viral escape [10]. Demonstration that RNAi expression cassettes under the control of the CMV promoter are effective paves the way for investigating use of other Pol II-driven cassettes that have properties of tissue-specific expression.

Human Factor VIII (FVIII) and alpha-1-antitrypsin (A1AT) promoters and HBV preS2 and core promoters are well-characterized liver-specific promoters and are potentially useful for specific expression of anti HBV pri-miR shuttles in liver tissue. The promoter of FVIII contains sequence elements that are recognized by the liver-enriched transcription factor hepatocyte nuclear factor 1 (HNF-1) [11].

Similarly liver-specific expression of the A1AT promoter is regulated by the liver transcription factors HNF-1α and HNF-4 [12]. Employing HBV regulatory elements for the liver-specific expression of pri-miR shuttle sequences is also appealing as the liver tropism exhibited by HBV is conferred in part by its transcription regulatory elements (reviewed in [6]).

Use of a pri-miR scaffold that is derived from the pri-miR-122 sequence that is abundantly expressed liver cells only [13] is also potentially useful for conferring liver specificity on antiviral RNAi activators. In this study, we report on the generation of liver-specific pri-miR-122-derived anti HBV shuttle expression cassettes that are capable of efficient viral gene silencing without evidence for disrupting the endogenous miR pathway.

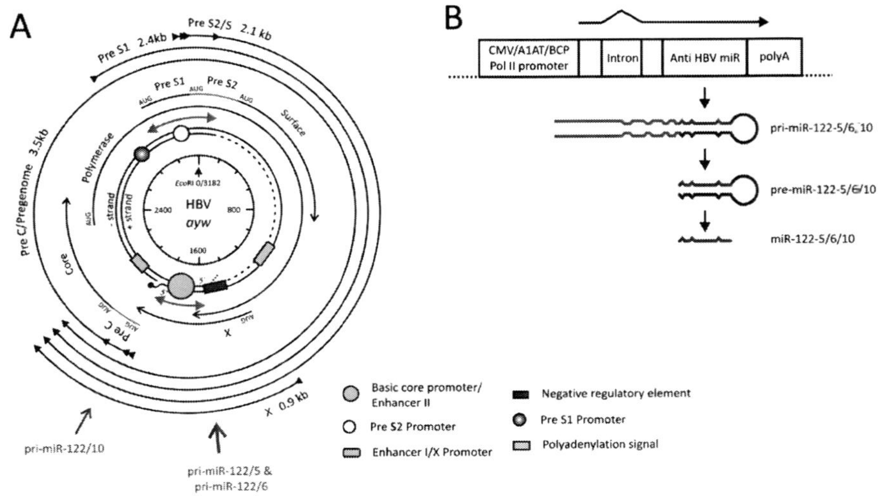

Figure 1. Organization HBV genome and Pol II antiviral expression cassettes. A. The partially double stranded circular genome with cis elements and coordinates calculated relative to the unique EcoRI restriction site are indicated at the center. Viral open reading frames are shown as arrows immediately surrounding the genome. The outermost arrows represent the four major viral transcripts that terminate at a single polyadenylation site. Sites within the *HBx* ORF that are targeted by the miR shuttles are indicated. The BCP and PreS2 promoter sequences that were incorporated into Pol II expression cassettes are shown as double headed arrows. B. Schematic illustration of pri-miR-122 shuttle expression cassettes showing upstream Pol II promoter (CMV, A1AT, FVIII, BCP or PreS2), intron and pri-miR mimic sequences with downstream transcription termination signal (poly A). Pre-miR shuttles were inserted in an exon and were flanked by 51 nt of pri-miR-122-derived sequences. The putative pre-miRs generated after Drosha/DGCR8 processing are indicated in color (purple and red) and the mature processed guide sequences that are selected after Dicer processing and strand selection by RISC are indicated in red only.

Materials and Methods

Plasmids encoding HBV target sequences, constitutively active reporters and miR-16 sponges. The pCH-9/3091 [14], pTZ-FLuc and pCH-FLuc [9], psiCHECK-miR-16T×7 and pU6 miR-16S×7 [10] and pCI-neo eGFP [15] vectors have been described before.

To generate pCMV FLuc, a vector that encodes Firefly luciferase under control of the CMV immediate early promoter, the Firefly luciferase-encoding DNA fragment was removed from pTZ-FLuc after XhoI and SpeI restriction and inserted into XhoI and XbaI sites of pCI-neo (Promega, WI, USA).

CMV Pol-II promoter driven pri-miR-122 shuttle expression cassettes. Anti HBV pri-miR-122 shuttle sequences were designed to target sites within the *HBx* ORF (accession number J02203.1). pri-miR-122/5 encodes a guide that is complementary to co-ordinates 1575-1597, pri-miR-122/6 targets co-ordinates 1580-1602 and pri-miR-122/10 targets co-ordinates 1863-1885 of HBV (Figure 1A). Construction of the CMV pri-miR-122/5 shuttle expression cassette has been described previously [8, 9]. Propagation of Pol II-driven pri-miR-122/6 and pri-miR-122/10 shuttle cassettes was carried out using a similar approach, which initially involved formation of pre-miR-encoding sequences by extension of partially complementary forward (F) and reverse (R) oligonucleotide primers. The complete pri-miR-encoding sequences were then constituted by PCR amplification of the pre-miR template and subsequently ligated to liver-specific Pol II promoters. All oligonucleotides were synthesized using standard phosphoramidite chemistry (Inqaba Biotech, South Africa). The oligonucleotide sequences were as follows: pre-miR-122/6 F: 5'- GAG TTT CCT TAG CAG AGC TGG TGC AGA GGT GAA GCG AAG TGC AGT CTA AAC AAT GCA CTT CG -3', pre-miR-122/6 R: 5'- GGA TTG CCT AGC AGT AGC TAG GTC AGA GGT TAA GCG AAG TGC ATT GTT TAG ACT GCA CTT CG -3', pre-miR-122/10 F: 5'- GAG TTT CCT TAG CAG AGC TGA GGC ACA GCT TGG AGG CTT GAA CGT CTA AAC TAT TTC AAG CC -3' and pre-miR-122/10 R: 5'- GGA TTG CCT AGC AGT AGC TAA TTC ACA GCT GGG AGG CTT GAA ATA GTT TAG ACG TTC AAG CC -3'. Purified products from primer extension were used as template in PCR using universal pri-miR-122 F (5'- GAC TGC TAG CTG GAG GTG AAG TTA ACA CCT TCG TGG CTA CAG AGT TTC CTT AGC AGA GCT G -3') and pri-miR-122 R (5'- GAT CAC TAG TAA AAA AGC AAA CGA TGC CAA GAC ATT TAT CGA GGG AAG GAT TGC CTA GCA GTA GCT A-3') primers. The pri-miR-122 shuttle fragments were ligated to the PCR cloning vector pTZ57R/T (InsTAclone™ PCR cloning Kit, Fermentas, MD, USA) according to the manufacturer's instructions to generate the pTZ-pri-miR-122 vectors. To generate CMV-driven pri-miR-122/6 and pri-miR-122/10 expression cassettes, the pri-miR-122/6 and pri-miR-122/10 shuttle sequences were excised from their respective pTZ vectors using NheI and XbaI and inserted into equivalent sites of pCI-neo (Promega, WI, USA). This procedure was similar to that previously described for propagating pCMV pri-miR-122/5 [9].

Liver-specific reporter and pri-miR-122 shuttle expression vectors. The human A1AT (Genbank accession number D38257.1) and FVIII (Genbank accession number NT_167198.1) promoter sequences were amplified from total human genomic DNA extracted from Huh7 cells using standard PCR procedures. Primers A1AT F (5'- GAT CTG ATC ATT CCC TGG TCT GAA TGT GTG -3') and A1AT R (5'- GAT CAA GCT TAC TGT CCC AGG TCA GTG GTG -3') were used to amplify the A1AT promoter. Similarly FVIII F (5'- GAT CAG ATC TGA GCT CAC CAT GGC TAC ATT -3') and FVIII R (5'- GAT CAA GCT TGA CTT ATT GCT ACA AAT GTT CAA C -3') generated a FVIII promoter sequence. The PCR amplicons extended from nucleotides 75856176 - 75854902 of chromosome 14 for the A1AT promoter sequence and nucleotides 5169940 - 5168766 of the X chromosome for the FVIII promoter sequence. The HBV Basic Core Promoter (BCP) and preS2 promoter sequences (Genbank accession number J02203.1) were amplified from the plasmid pCH-9/3091 using the following primer sets: BCP F (5'- GAT CAG ATC TGC ATG GAG ACC ACC GTG AAC -3'), BCP R (5'- GAT CAA GCT TCA CCC AAG GCA CAG CTT GGA -3'), PreS2 F (5'- GAT CAG ATC TGC CTT CAG AGC AAA CAC CGC -3') and PreS2 R (5'- GAT CAA GCT TAC AGG CCT CTC ACT CTG GGA -3'). Amplicons extended from viral nucleotide coordinates 1606 to 1890 for BCP and from 2911 - 50 for the PreS2 promoter (Figure 1A). All oligonucleotides were synthesized by standard phosphoramidite chemistry (Inqaba Biotech, South Africa). Primers were designed such that amplification introduced a BglII (BclI in the case of A1AT) site at the 5' end and a HindIII site at the 3' end of the amplicons. PCR was carried out using the Expand High Fidelity PCR^{PLUS} System (Roche Diagnostics GmbH, Germany) according to manufacturer's instructions. Purified amplicons were ligated to the linearized PCR cloning vector pTZ57R/T to generate pTZ-A1AT, pTZ-FVIII, pTZ-BCP and pTZ-PreS2. Positive plasmid clones were identified using restriction enzyme mapping and sequences were verified using standard automated dideoxy chain termination procedures (Inqaba Biotech, South Africa).

To generate liver-specific Pol II expression plasmids, the CMV immediate early enhancer promoter transcriptional regulatory element within pCI-neo (Promega, WI, USA) was substituted with the sequences of the liver-specific promoters. The sequences encoding the FVIII, BCP and PreS2 promoter elements were removed from pTZ-FVIII, pTZ-BCP and pTZ-PreS2 using

BglII and HindIII restriction and the A1AT sequence was excised from pTZ-A1AT using BclI and HindIII. Since BclI is sensitive to methylation, pTZ-A1AT was propagated in the dcm- and dam-methylase deficient strain of *E. coli*, GM2929. pCI-neo was digested with HindIII and EcoRI to yield 3815 bp, 1317 bp and 340 bp fragments. Separately, pCI-neo was digested with EcoRI and BglII to yield 4371 and 1101 bp fragments. Liver-specific promoter sequences were ligated with the 340 bp HindIII-EcoRI and the 4371 bp EcoRI-BglII fragments in a three-way ligation reaction to generate backbone liver-specific expression vectors (pA1AT, pFVIII, pBCP and pPreS2). BclI and BglII generated complementary overhangs thus allowing the A1AT promoter sequence to be ligated to the pCI-neo backbone. These plasmids contained the liver-specific promoter sequences followed by a chimeric intron and an SV40 late polyadenylation signal downstream of the insert (Figure 1B).

To generate Pol II reporter gene expression cassettes, the Firefly luciferase sequence was removed from pCMV FLuc [9] after digestion with NheI and SmaI then ligated to equivalent sites of the liver-specific expression vectors to generate pA1AT FLuc, pFVIII FLuc, pBCP FLuc and pPreS2 FLuc. Plasmids containing liver-specific pri-miR-122-derived cassettes were propagated after ligation of pri-miR-122 shuttles, excised from pCMV pri-miR-122/5, pCMV pri-miR-122/6 and pCMV pri-miR-122/10 using NheI and SmaI, to equivalent sites of pA1AT and pBCP.

Cell Culture. Functionality of liver-specific expression cassettes was assessed in Huh7 cells and the HEK293-derived 116 cells by co-transfecting 100 ng of each of the different Pol II Firefly luciferase expression vectors, 100 ng of phRL-CMV (Promega, WI, USA) and 100 ng of pCI-neo eGFP. Transfection was achieved using Lipofectamine™ 2000 (Invitrogen, CA, USA) according to manufacturer's instructions. Firefly and *Renilla* luciferase activities were assayed using the Dual-Luciferase® Assay System (Promega, WI, USA) and measured on a Veritas Dual Injection Luminometer (Turner BioSystems, CA, USA). Firefly luciferase activity was normalized to *Renilla* luciferase activity. Detection of Firefly luciferase activity that was exclusive to the liver-derived cell line was interpreted as liver-specific expression. To assess the tissue-specificity of silencing by the liver-specific pri-miR shuttles, Huh7 and 116 cells were transfected with 80 ng of target plasmid (pCH-FLuc). Together with this plasmid, 800 ng of the A1AT- and BCP-driven pri-miR shuttle vectors, 50 ng of phRL-CMV and 50 ng of pCI-neo eGFP were also transfected. Plasmid DNA was made up to a total of 1 μg with pCI-neo (Promega, WI, USA) and transfected as described above. Forty eight hours post-transfection cells were lysed and measurement of Firefly and *Renilla* luciferase activities was carried out.

Possible disruption of the miR biogenesis pathway by the A1AT and BCP Pri-miR-122 shuttle expression cassettes was assessed in Huh7 cells after co-transfecting RNAi effecter expression cassettes and the miR-16 target vector, psiCHECK-miR-16T×7. This assay, an adaptation of the use of miR sponges to derepress miR function [16], has been described previously [10]. Cells were co-transfected with 80 ng of psiCHECK-miR-16T×7, 800 ng of RNAi effecter or sponge (pU6-miR-16S×7) vectors and 120 ng of pCI-neo eGFP using Lipofectamine™ 2000.

Assessing efficacy in vivo of liver-specific pri-miR shuttle sequences. In vivo efficacy of the A1AT- and BCP-driven pri-miR-122 shuttle expression cassettes was further assessed by employing the hydrodynamic injection model of HBV replication.

Five micrograms of liver-specific anti HBV expression cassettes were co-injected with 5 μg each of pCH-9/3091 and pCI-neo eGFP. Blood samples were collected from mice 3 and 5 days post-injection and HBsAg concentrations determined using the MONOLISA® HBs Ag Assay kit (Bio-Rad, CA, USA). All procedures were carried out in accordance with protocols approved by the Animal Ethics Screening Committee of the University of the Witwatersrand.

Statistical Analysis. The student's t-test was carried out to determine statistical significance and this was determined using the GraphPad Prism Software version 4.03 (GraphPad Software, CA, USA).

Results

Selection of liver-specific Pol II promoters for expression of pri-miR shuttle cassettes. Initially, to establish whether the selected promoter sequences are functional and exhibit tissue-specificity, the ability of these transcriptional elements to express the Firefly luciferase reporter gene was assessed.

This was determined by quantitation of Firefly luciferase activity in human liver-derived (Huh7) and non hepatic human kidney-derived (115) cells. Sequences spanning nucleotides -1175 to -9 upstream of the *FVIII* [17] gene and nucleotides -1200 to -32 upstream of the *A1AT* [18] gene have been shown to drive transcription of reporter genes in liver-derived cell lines and were included in the expression cassettes used here.

Plasmids expressing the reporter gene from a CMV immediate early promoter enhancer element (pCMV FLuc) and each from the panel of putative liver-specific Pol II promoters (pA1AT FLuc, pFVIII FLuc, pBCP FLuc and pPreS2 FLuc) were used to transfect cells in culture. Firefly luciferase was strongly expressed in both Huh7 and 116 cells after transfection with pCMV FLuc (Figure 2). This is not unexpected as the CMV immediate early promoter enhancer is known to be ubiquitously active and powerful [19].

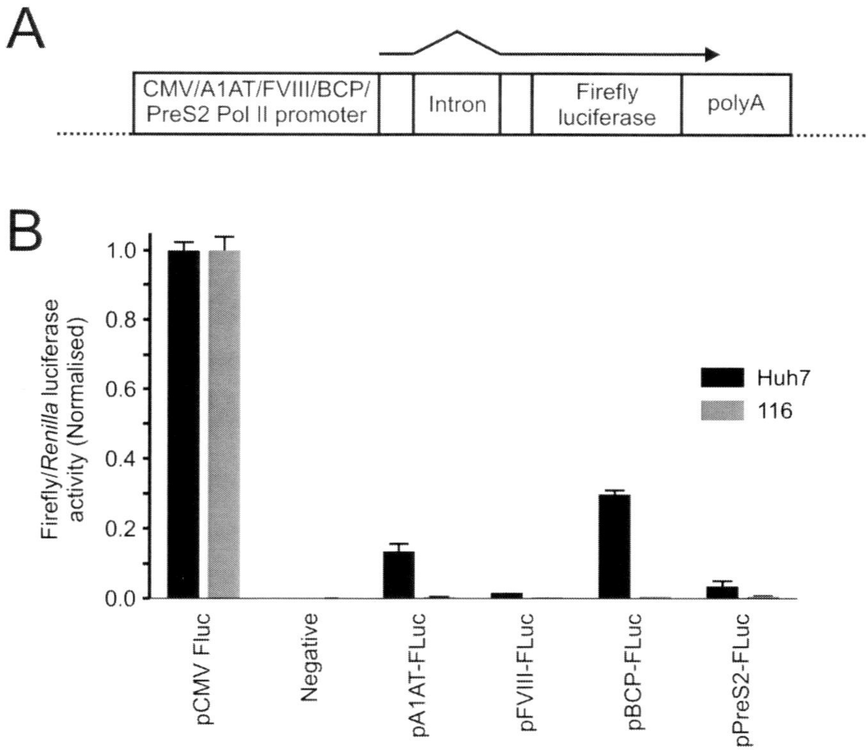

Figure 2. Reporter gene assay to determine liver specificity of Pol II promoters. A. Schematic illustration of the structure of the Pol II expression cassettes encoding the Firefly luciferase reporter. B. Functionality and tissue-specificity of the putative liver-specific promoters was assessed by measuring expression of the Firefly luciferase activity in liver-derived (Huh7) and kidney-derived (116) cells. Bars indicate means of relative Firefly to Renilla luciferase activity in Huh7 (black bars) and 116 (gray bars) cells. Error bars indicate standard error of the mean (SEM).

Measurement of Firefly luciferase activity in Huh7 cells that were transfected with the liver-specific expression plasmids indicated that these promoter sequences were functional. In contrast to the expression from the CMV immediate early promoter enhancer Firefly luciferase activity was not detected in kidney-derived cells when expressed from any of the liver-specific promoters, which indicated that these cassettes exhibit tissue-specific expression. However, reporter gene activity derived from expression of the CMV promoter sequence was significantly stronger than that of the other liver-specific promoters. FVIII and PreS2 promoters showed very low activity, which was unlikely to achieve sufficient pri-miR shuttle expression, and were excluded from additional investigation. To advance the analysis of expression of anti HBV shuttles from liver specific Pol II promoters, CMV, A1AT and BCP transcriptional regulatory elements were selected for further study. A total of nine pri-miR-122 shuttle Pol II expression cassettes were then tested for silencing of HBV replication in cell culture and in vivo. These were the pri-miR-122/5, pri-miR-122/6 and pri-miR-122/10 shuttle sequences, which were each placed under transcriptional control of the CMV, A1AT or BCP promoters (Figure 1B).

Pri-miR shuttle sequences driven from the A1AT and HBV core promoters are capable of inhibiting HBV replication in cultured liver-derived cells. Tissue-specific expression achieved by the A1AT and HBV core promoter sequences indicated that these sequences would be useful for expression of anti HBV pri-miR-122 shuttles. To asses this, silencing of the HBV target was initially determined using a reporter gene plasmid (pCH-FLuc) that allowed sensitive and quantitative assessment of HBV targeting in situ. In pCH-FLuc, the preS2/S sequence of pCH-9/3091 [14] was replaced with the Firefly luciferase ORF and the targeted HBx ORF remained intact (Figure 3A).

Results show that pri-miR-122/5 shuttle sequences expressed from the CMV promoter caused knockdown of HBV gene expression in liver- and kidney-derived cell lines (Figure 3B).

However, equivalent knockdown by the A1AT and BCP shuttle vector was only achieved in the liver-derived cell line. Knockdown in the kidney-derived cell line by the tissue-specific pri-miR shuttle vectors was minimal and significantly lower than the silencing achieved by the CMV pri-miR shuttles. Interestingly CMV pri-miR-122/6 did not cause significant silencing in the kidney-derived cell line, which is likely to be a result of lower efficacy of the pri-miR-122/6 sequence.

The pri-miR-122/10 shuttle, which is known to be ineffective against HBV [8, 9], was incapable of reporter knockdown irrespective of the promoter from which it was expressed. CMV pri-miR-122/10 seemed to induce HBV expression and is in accordance with previous observations using a similar guide incorporated into U6 short hairpin RNA cassette (U6 shRNA 10) [8].

Collectively these data indicate that anti HBV pri-miR shuttle sequences retain their silencing capabilities when expressed from liver-specific promoters. The silencing activity by A1AT- and BCP-pri-miR-122/5 expression cassettes, which is limited to liver-derived cell lines, prompted investigation of their efficacy in vivo.

A1AT-driven pri-miR shuttle sequences knock down a marker of HBV replication in vivo. Efficacy in vivo of the A1AT- and BCP-driven pri-miR shuttle expression cassettes was assessed using the hydrodynamic injection model of HBV replication. After co injecting animals with an HBV replication competent plasmid together with pri-miR expression cassettes, serum HBsAg concentrations were measured at days 3 and 5 post-injection (Figure 3C).

Assay of this viral antigen is a useful marker of viral replication and may be used to assess HBV knockdown [8]. No silencing of HBV replication was observed in mice that received BCP-driven pri-miR-122 shuttle expression cassettes and may reflect poor activity of this transcriptional control element in murine hepatocytes [20].

Silencing was achieved with pA1AT pri-miR-122/5 and was initially equivalent to that of its CMV promoter-driven counterpart. However, knockdown efficacy with plasmids containing the liver-specific transcription control element to express miR shuttles was not as durable as that achieved with the CMV expression cassettes.

This observation may be explained by the relative strengths of the A1AT and CMV promoters. The A1AT promoter is considerably weaker than the CMV promoter (Figure 2).

After hydrodynamic injection, plasmids transfect hepatocytes transiently. With time, a decrease in the intracellular concentration of pA1AT pri-miR-122/5 will result in a lower antiviral RNAi effecter concentration with concomitant diminished antiviral efficacy. Nevertheless this result demonstrates that weaker liver-specific promoters have potential use for therapeutic application and emphasizes the importance of utilizing exogenous RNAi activators that are effective at low concentrations. However, excluding the potentially harmful effects of derangement of the endogenous miR pathway is important.

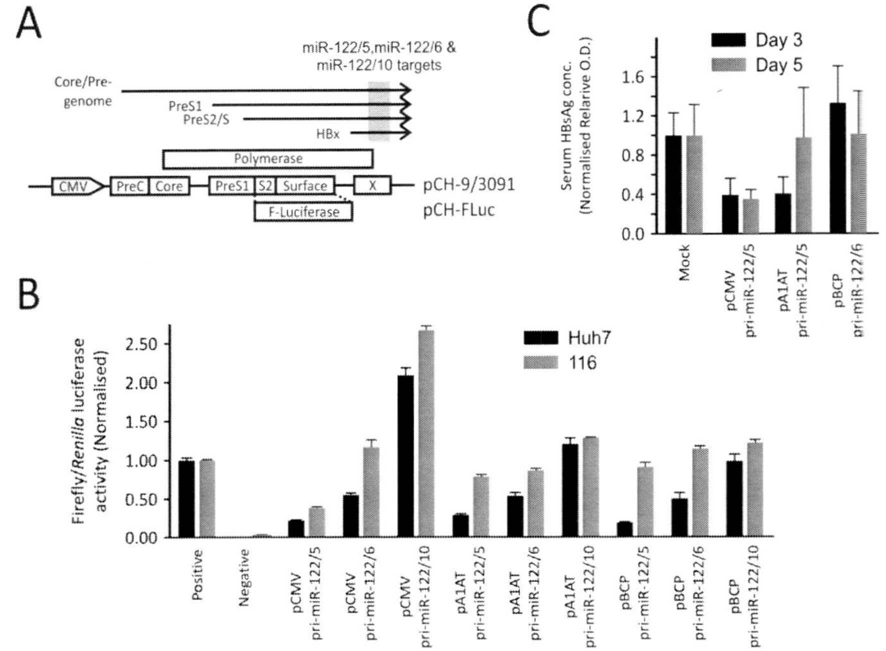

Figure 3. Inhibitory activity in cultured cells and in vivo of pri-miR-122 shuttle sequences expressed from various Pol II transcriptional regulatory elements. A. Organization of the HBV genome with ORFs and sites within the pCH-9/3091 vector that are targets complementary to anti HBV pri-miR-122 shuttles are shown. Four parallel arrows indicate the HBV transcripts, which have common 3′ ends, and include the pri-miR-122/5, pri-miR-122/6 and pri-miR-122/10 targets. The pCH-9/3091-derived pCH-FLuc target vector has the *Firefly luciferase* ORF substituted for the preS2/S HBV sequence. B. Anti HBV efficacy of liver-specific pri-miR-122 shuttles was assessed by co-transfection of Huh7 and 116 cells with pCH-FLuc and the various Pol II expression cassettes. Bars indicate means of relative Firefly to *Renilla* luciferase activities from Huh7 (black bars) and 116 (grey bars) cells. Error bars indicate SEM. C. Silencing of HBV replication *in vivo*. Serum concentration of HBsAg was measured at days 3 and 5 after hydrodynamic injection of mice with pCH-9/3091 and plasmids expressing anti HBV RNAi sequences. Mock injections included the control backbone plasmid containing the CMV promoter without anti HBV RNAi effecters. Each group comprised at least 4 mice and serum was collected 3 and 5 days after injection. HBsAg concentrations were determined by ELISA and mean concentrations of the viral antigen are indicated with SEM.

Liver-specific pri-miR-122 shuttle expression cassettes do not disrupt silencing of a reporter target by endogenous miR-16. To assess whether the liver-specific pri-miR-122 shuttle expression cassettes cause disruption of the miR biogenesis pathway, the previously described miR-16 saturation assay was carried out [10]. This assay is based on the use of miR sponges to derepress miR function [16]. Co-transfection of the control miR-16 sponge plasmid with a plasmid containing a miR-16 downstream of the Renilla *luciferase* ORF (Figure 4A), caused derepression of reporter activity when compared to mock-transfected cells (Figure 4B).

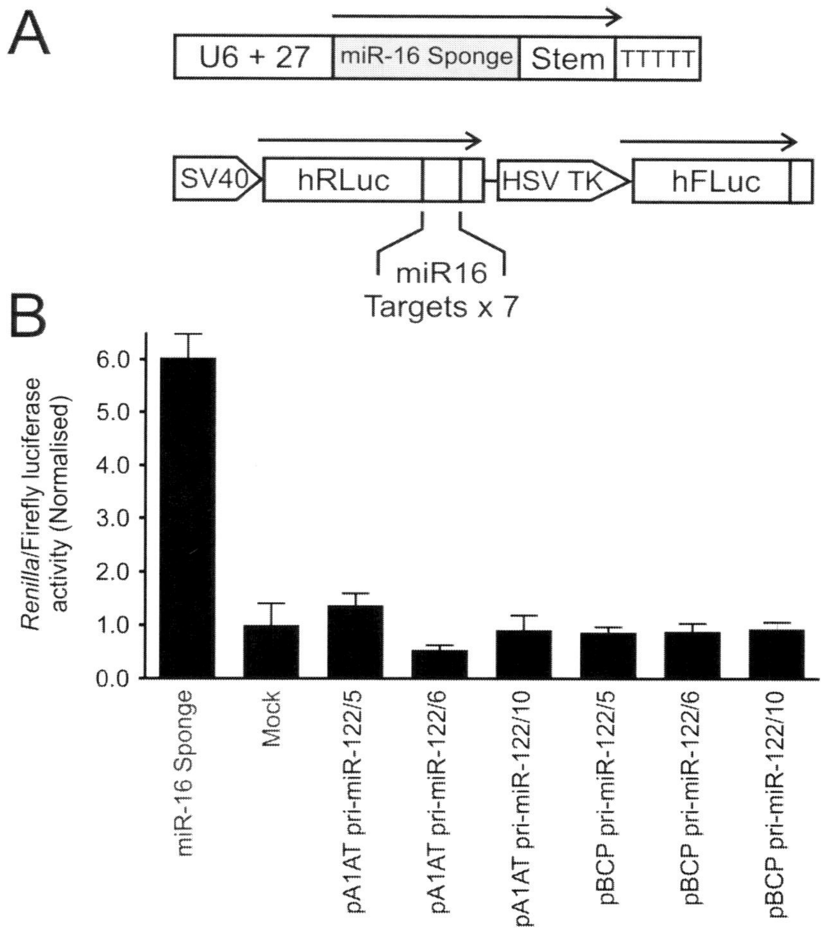

Figure 4. *Assessing saturation of the miR biogenesis pathway by miR-122 shuttles.*
A. Schematic representation of the sponge and psiCHECK-miR-16T×7 target plasmids. The dual luciferase reporter target expresses the Renilla *luciferase* transcript with miR-16 target sites within the 3' UTR, and also the untargeted *Firefly luciferase* ORF as normalizing control. B. Huh7 cells were co-transfected with the indicated plasmids and psiCHECK-miR-16T×7 in triplicate and the cells analyzed for luciferase activity 48 hours later. Means of the relative *Renilla* to Firefly luciferase activity are indicated with SEM.

This result accords with previous observations and verified that the sponge plasmid interfered with endogenous miR-16 silencing of the Renilla *luciferase* target. In contrast, none of the liver-specific pri-miR shuttle sequence expression cassettes derepressed *Renilla* luciferase activity, indicating that they do not disrupt endogenous miR-16 function. This result is not unexpected. The CMV immediate early promoter enhancer is a more powerful transcriptional control element than the liver-specific promoters (Figure 2), and miR shuttles expressed from the CMV promoter have previously been shown to have little effect on the endogenous miR biogenesis pathway [9, 10]. Lower amounts of pri-miR shuttle sequences should be transcribed from the liver-specific promoters, and are therefore unlikely to outcompete naturally occurring miR for processing by the RNAi processing machinery.

Discussion

Until recently Pol II promoter-regulated RNAi expression cassettes have been characterized by variable efficacy and utility [21-23]. Some of their limitations may be ascribed to difficulties with processing of traditional shRNA sequences that are transcribed from Pol II promoters. The subsequent development of pre- and pri-miR shuttle sequences as RNAi effecters has allowed improved transcription control by exploiting the natural miR biogenesis pathway. pri-miRs are typically transcribed from Pol II regulatory elements and expression of pri-miR shuttle sequences may therefore be subjected to control by these transcription regulatory elements. In support of this, we have previously shown that embedding anti HBV guides within RNAi effecters that mimic naturally occurring pri-miRs enable these sequences to be transcribed from Pol II promoters without compromising silencing activity [9, 10].

In the study reported here, we have extended this observation by demonstrating that miR-122 shuttle sequences may be controlled by liver-specific Pol II promoter elements. However, although efficient and sustained knockdown was achieved in cultured mammalian cells, silencing in vivo was not maintained for longer than 3 days. A likely reason for this observation is that the liver-specific Pol II regulatory elements described here are weaker than the CMV element.

Diminished expression of pri-miR shuttles, which accompanies the decreasing number of intrahepatocyte plasmid copies after transient hydrodynamic transfection, is associated with an attenuation of silencing efficacy that is more marked than that observed with the stronger CMV promoter. Improving promoter strength of liver-specific Pol II expression cassettes is therefore a priority of developing this approach. To achieve this, it may be necessary to combine transcription cis elements to optimize promoter strength and liver specificity.

By combining a murine alpha-fetoprotein enhancer with a minimal albumin promoter sequence this approach was recently reported to improve expression of an antiviral RNAi activator [24]. The natural propensity for certain miRs to be expressed abundantly in the liver, such as miR-122, indicate that transcription control of these silencing sequences may also be utilized to achieve liver-specific production of anti HBV RNAi activators.

A further refinement of tissue-specific expression of anti HBV miRs would be their production from cassettes that are induced following viral infection. HBV encodes a promiscuous trans activator, HBx, that is capable of indirect induction of transcription through interaction with a variety of trans factors (reviewed in [25]).

Incorporating Pol II promoter elements into anti HBV miR expression cassettes that are sensitive and responsive to HBx would be an interesting approach that could further improve regulation of expression of antiviral sequences. An alternative approach is to use regulatory elements that may be controlled by administration or withdrawal of drugs. The recently describe steroid-inducible liver-specific promoter is such an example that could be used to control pri-miR shuttle expression [26].

Tight transcriptional control is important to limit toxic effects of potentially therapeutic exogenous RNAi activators. Unwanted effects, such as silencing of essential cellular sequences and disruption of the natural miR pathway, are more likely to arise as a result of off target and uncontrolled expression of RNAi effecter sequences. To achieve optimal specific silencing, it is also critically important to select RNAi effecter sequences that are potent, that is effective at low concentrations.

A therapeutic sequence that is effective against its target at low concentration is less likely to cause unwanted side effects. Expression of potent pri-miR shuttle sequences from regulatable promoters is therefore required to achieve a balance between the required effective concentration of silencing sequences and avoidance of off target effects.

The present study advances this approach and further supports the potential therapeutic utility of tissue-specific Pol II-expressed pri-miR shuttle expression cassettes.

Acknowledgments

Work in the authors' laboratory is supported by funding from the Sixth Research Framework Programme of the European Union, Project RIGHT (LSHB-CT-2004-005276), CANSA, the South African National Research Foundation (NRF GUN 68339 and 65495), ESASTAP and the South African Poliomyelitis Research Foundation.

References

[1] WHO. Hepatitis B virus Fact sheet No. 204 (Revised 2008). 2000; Available from: http://www.who.int/mediacentre/factsheets/fs204/en/index.html.

[2] Lee, W.M., Hepatitis B virus infection. *N. Engl. J. Med.*, 1997. 337(24): p. 1733-45.

[3] Arbuthnot, P. and M. Kew, Hepatitis B virus and hepatocellular carcinoma. *Int. J. Exp. Pathol.,* 2001. 82(2): p. 77-100.

[4] Chien, Y.C., et al., Nationwide hepatitis B vaccination program in Taiwan: effectiveness in the 20 years after it was launched. *Epidemiol. Rev.,* 2006. 28: p. 126-35.

[5] Karayiannis, P., Hepatitis B virus: old, new and future approaches to antiviral treatment. *J. Antimicrob. Chemother.,* 2003. 51(4): p. 761-85.

[6] Moolla, N., M. Kew, and P. Arbuthnot, Regulatory elements of hepatitis B virus transcription. *Journal of Viral Hepatitis,* 2002. 9(5): p. 323-331.

[7] Seeger, C., D. Ganem, and H.E. Varmus, Biochemical and genetic evidence for the hepatitis B virus replication strategy. *Science,* 1986. 232(4749): p. 477-84.

[8] Carmona, S., et al., Effective inhibition of HBV replication in vivo by anti-HBx short hairpin RNAs. *Mol. Ther.,* 2006. 13(2): p. 411-21.

[9] Ely, A., et al., Expressed anti-HBV primary microRNA shuttles inhibit viral replication efficiently in vitro and in vivo. *Mol. Ther.,* 2008. 16(5): p. 1105-12.

[10] Ely, A., T. Naidoo, and P. Arbuthnot, Efficient silencing of gene expression with modular trimeric Pol II expression cassettes comprising microRNA shuttles. *Nucleic Acids Research*, 2009. 37(13): p. e91.

[11] McGlynn, L.K., et al., Role of the liver-enriched transcription factor hepatocyte nuclear factor 1 in transcriptional regulation of the factor V111 gene. *Mol. Cell Biol.,* 1996. 16(5): p. 1936-45.
[12] Kalsheker, N., S. Morley, and K. Morgan, Gene regulation of the serine proteinase inhibitors alpha1-antitrypsin and alpha1-antichymotrypsin. *Biochem. Soc. Trans.,* 2002. 30(2): p. 93-8.
[13] Chang, J., et al., miR-122, a mammalian liver-specific microRNA, is processed from hcr mRNA and may downregulate the high affinity cationic amino acid transporter CAT-1. *RNA Biol.,* 2004. 1(2): p. 106-13.
[14] Nassal, M., The arginine-rich domain of the hepatitis B virus core protein is required for pregenome encapsidation and productive viral positive-strand DNA synthesis but not for virus assembly. *J. Virol.,* 1992. 66(7): p. 4107-16.
[15] Passman, M., et al., In situ demonstration of inhibitory effects of hammerhead ribozymes that are targeted to the hepatitis Bx sequence in cultured cells. *Biochem. Biophys. Res. Commun.,* 2000. 268(3): p. 728-33.
[16] Ebert, M.S., J.R. Neilson, and P.A. Sharp, MicroRNA sponges: competitive inhibitors of small RNAs in mammalian cells. *Nat. Methods,* 2007. 4(9): p. 721-6.
[17] Figueiredo, M.S. and G.G. Brownlee, cis-acting elements and transcription factors involved in the promoter activity of the human factor VIII gene. *J. Biol. Chem.,* 1995. 270(20): p. 11828-38.
[18] Ciliberto, G., L. Dente, and R. Cortese, Cell-specific expression of a transfected human alpha 1-antitrypsin gene. *Cell,* 1985. 41(2): p. 531-40.
[19] Schmidt, E.V., et al., The cytomegalovirus enhancer: a pan-active control element in transgenic mice. *Mol. Cell Biol.,* 1990. 10(8): p. 4406-11.
[20] 2Rih, J., et al., The Action of Hepatitis B Virus Enhancer 2-Core Gene Promoter in Non-Viral and Retroviral Vectors for Hepatocyte-Specific Expression. *J. Biochem. Mol. Biol.,* 1997. 30: p. 269-273.
[21] Peng, Y., J.X. Lu, and X.F. Shen, shRNA driven by Pol II/T7 dual-promoter system effectively induce cell-specific RNA interference in mammalian cells. *Biochem. Biophys. Res. Commun.,* 2007. 360(2): p. 496-500.
[22] Yuan, J., et al., shRNA transcribed by RNA Pol II promoter induce RNA interference in mammalian cell. *Mol. Biol. Rep.,* 2006. 33(1): p. 43-9.

[23] Giering, J.C., et al., Expression of shRNA from a tissue-specific pol II promoter is an effective and safe RNAi therapeutic. *Mol. Ther.,* 2008. 16(9): p. 1630-6.

[24] Snyder, L.L., et al., Vector design for liver-specific expression of multiple interfering RNAs that target hepatitis B virus transcripts. *Antiviral. Res.,* 2008. 80(1): p. 36-44.

[25] Arbuthnot, P., A. Capovilla, and M. Kew, Putative role of hepatitis B virus X protein in hepatocarcinogenesis: effects on apoptosis, DNA repair, mitogen-activated protein kinase and JAK/STAT pathways. *J. Gastroenterol. Hepatol.,* 2000. 15(4): p. 357-68.

[26] Wang, L., et al., Prolonged and inducible transgene expression in the liver using gutless adenovirus: a potential therapy for liver cancer. *Gastroenterology,* 2004. 126(1): p. 278-289.

Index

A

D

H

I

J

K

L

M

N

O

P

R

S

T

U

V

W

X

Y